The Opioid Epidemic and the Therapeutic Community Model

Jonathan D. Avery
Kristopher A. Kast
Editors

The Opioid Epidemic and the Therapeutic Community Model

An Essential Guide

Springer

Editors
Jonathan D. Avery
Weill Cornell Medical College
New York, NY
USA

Kristopher A. Kast
Payne Whitney Clinic of
New York-Presbyterian
Weill Cornell Medical College
New York, NY
USA

ISBN 978-3-030-26272-3   ISBN 978-3-030-26273-0 (eBook)
https://doi.org/10.1007/978-3-030-26273-0

This Springer imprint is published by the registered company Springer Nature Switzerland AG
The registered company address is: Gewerbestrasse 11, 6330 Cham, Switzerland

Acknowledgments

The authors would like to thank Daniele Bodini, the Alexander Bodini Foundation, and Friends of San Patrignano, USA, for their support of this work.

Contents

1 **An Introduction to the Opioid Epidemic and Therapeutic Communities** 1
Kristopher A. Kast and Jonathan D. Avery

2 **Therapeutic Communities: Evolutionary Arc and the Opioid Epidemic** 9
George De Leon

3 **The Modern Therapeutic Community Model** 23
Fernando B. Perfas

4 **The Opioid Epidemic** 45
Rachel Knight

5 **Response to the Opioid Epidemic: Current Treatment Models in the United States**. 63
Joseph Bravoco

6 **Target Population: Treatment-Resistant Opioid Use Disorder and the Role of Therapeutic Communities** 75
Kristopher A. Kast

7 **Current Therapeutic Communities Around the World** 87
Phaedon Kaloterakis

8 Therapeutic Communities and the Judicial System in the United States 113
Andrew Tuck and Lauren Stossel

9 San Patrignano: Lessons from the Italian Experience 133
Gabriele Manella, Giovanni Pieretti, Alessandra Landi, and Bruno Genetti

Index 149

Contributors

Jonathan D. Avery, MD Weill Cornell Medical College, New York, NY, USA

Joseph Bravoco New York-Presbyterian Hospital/Weill Cornell Medical Center, New York, NY, USA

George De Leon Department of Psychiatry, New York University School of Medicine, New York, NY, USA

Bruno Genetti Centro Studi Explora, Padua, Italy

Phaedon Kaloterakis KETHEA, European Federation of Therapeutic Communities (EFTC), World Federation of Therapeutic Communities (WFTC), Thessaloniki, Greece

Kristopher A. Kast, MD Payne Whitney Clinic of New York-Presbyterian, Weill Cornell Medical College, New York, NY, USA

Rachel Knight, MD New York Presbyterian – Weill Cornell Medical Center, New York, NY, USA

Alessandra Landi Department of Sociology and Business Law, University of Bologna, Bologna, Italy

Gabriele Manella Department of Sociology and Business Law, University of Bologna, Bologna, Italy

Fernando B. Perfas, PhD Addiction Training Consultant, Red Hook, NY, USA

Giovanni Pieretti Department of Sociology and Business Law, University of Bologna, Bologna, Italy

Lauren Stossel, MD Correctional Health Services, NYC Health+Hospitals, New York, NY, USA

Andrew Tuck, BS Columbia University Vagelos College of Physicians & Surgeons, New York, NY, USA

An Introduction to the Opioid Epidemic and Therapeutic Communities

1

Kristopher A. Kast and Jonathan D. Avery

The Opioid Epidemic

Opioids have been written into our contemporary American zeitgeist, overflowing the prescription pads that have flooded medicine cabinets and illicit marketplaces with up to 80 scripts per 100 persons at the peak of the crisis we have collectively faced since the turn of the twenty-first century [19].

In 2017, 4.2% of the United States' general population has been exposed to opioids in a way not directed by a prescribing clinician—including use without a prescription and use in greater amounts, more often, or for longer periods than directed [16]. Of the 11.4 million Americans in this group, 2.5 million have an opioid use disorder (OUD) [16]. Individuals with OUD experience significant medical and functional sequelae, with markedly increased rates of emergency medical service utilization, infectious disease complications (including human

K. A. Kast (✉)
Payne Whitney Clinic of New York-Presbyterian,
Weill Cornell Medical College, New York, NY, USA
e-mail: kak9100@nyp.org

J. D. Avery
Weill Cornell Medical College, New York, NY, USA
e-mail: joa9070@med.cornell.edu

J. D. Avery, K. A. Kast (eds.), *The Opioid Epidemic and the Therapeutic Community Model*, https://doi.org/10.1007/978-3-030-26273-0_1

immunodeficiency virus and viral hepatitides), obstetrics and neonatal complications in mothers with OUD and their newborns, impaired social and occupational functioning, legal system involvement, homelessness, and death [18].

In the United States, OUD and its associated morbidity and mortality have received increasing attention from national public health authorities, medical professional organizations, federal and local government, and the lay press over the past decade. Contemporary OUD is most commonly associated with prescription opioid use—now threefold more frequent than OUD associated with heroin use—and prescription opioid overdose deaths have quadrupled between 1999 and 2011, continuing to rise to a peak of 72,000 total drug overdose deaths per year in 2017.

This "opioid epidemic," or crisis, has motivated a series of federal responses, including the Comprehensive Addiction and Recovery Act (CARA) of 2016 [8, 9, 14, 16]. CARA's implementation has emphasized increasing access to currently underutilized medication-assisted treatment (or MAT, including methadone, buprenorphine, and naltrexone formulations) alongside naloxone-based and other harm-reduction measures against overdose deaths. These are evidence-based interventions with proven efficacy in reducing relapse and OUD-related death, OUD-related infectious disease transmission, criminal recidivism, as well as increasing treatment retention [8, 12, 13, 20]. Despite this evidence base, only a minority of patients receive appropriate MAT, and efforts to increase access to these interventions are much needed [8, 11].

However, a significant group continues opioid use with its grave risks despite these first-line treatments, marking a population with treatment-resistant opioid use disorder for whom additional interventions are required. For some patients, relative medical contraindications or aversions to one or all of the available medications also limit their ability to benefit from MAT.

Further, the current system of care wherein MAT is delivered emphasizes short-term rehabilitation, with 30- or 60-day lengths of stay (LOS) being most common. This is problematic for the treatment-resistant population in light of the multiply-replicated finding that greater LOS improves substance use-related outcomes—with a likely inflection point at 90 days and continued benefit with even longer treatment for more severely impaired individuals [2, 5, 6, 17].

Therapeutic Communities

The therapeutic community (TC) is a treatment modality that addresses OUD via mechanisms of action that differ from MAT and other common interventions currently available in the United States—including longer LOS, cognitive schema change, increased mentalization capacity, social learning, and educational/occupational habilitation. TCs may either complement current standards of care or serve as monotherapy for patients with severe, treatment-refractory OUD [3–5, 7, 15, 22, 23]. TCs have been effective in leading to sustained remission for OUD patients with significant markers of poor prognosis, including multiple substance use disorders, psychiatric comorbidity, personality disorder, poor work history, and criminality—a group difficult to study and often excluded from typical randomized-controlled trials of MAT and related interventions [4, 5].

Therapeutic communities for addiction arose in the United States in the late 1950s and early 1960s out of the peer-led 12-step tradition of Alcoholics Anonymous [10]. The first communities, Synanon and Daytop Village, emerged outside traditional healthcare systems; in fact, these early TCs have been identified both as an "alternative" to medical models of addiction treatment and as a part of the larger "anti-psychiatry" movement in the United States [1]. This in part explains the historical strict avoidance of psychotropic medications in TCs; the early abstinence-based model extended beyond alcohol and illicit drugs—it included mind-altering medications for psychiatric disorders, which were only beginning to be developed in the 1950s–1960s, with the first antidepressants and antipsychotics.

Methadone maintenance therapy, which was being studied for the treatment of OUD at the Rockefeller Institute in 1964, was initially viewed as a threat to sobriety and recovery by those in the early TC model. This historical perspective has been challenged with some difficulty, as the first study to ask if patients taking methadone can be successfully treated within a therapeutic community model was published relatively recently in 2009 [22].

Although traditionally espousing abstinence-based recovery, increasingly TCs incorporate MAT and other evidence-based treatments—including cognitive behavioral therapy, motivational interviewing, and relapse-prevention approaches—into treatment plans for patients [4, 5, 22]. Modern TCs are integrating into the overall system of care for addicted patients, with many now offering expanded services in primary medical care, mental health care, relapse-prevention training, and aftercare case management [5, 24].

The core therapeutic approach is simply "community as method," meaning the purposeful use of a complex social structure to teach patients to use the community to change themselves [5]. The structure of the TC has evolved over the decades, with many modifications in response to differing patient populations (including pregnant women, adolescents, and prisoners) and increasing fiscal pressure to shorten length of stay (LOS) from the original 12–24 months' duration.

TCs uniformly provide a stable residence in shared communal spaces that are separated from the prior drug-associated environment. They require urine toxicological screening and surveillance for all members. LOS is purposefully long term, ranging from 3 to 36 months, and is individualized to each community member. The community has a clear social structure, including peer and professional staff (typically, ~50% peer based) who serve to facilitate the planned community organization. Participation in structured community-enhancing activities for meals, work, therapeutic groups, celebration, and leisure is asked of each individual.

The model intensifies social learning, using participation in regular peer encounter groups with corrective "pull-ups" and affirming "push-ups" from peers to shape behavior toward shared community values and "right living." Additional behavioral feedback occurs via privileges earned to reward progression in the program and disciplinary sanctions for violations of rules protecting patient and staff safety and program culture. There are also straightforward educational seminars around the fundamental philosophy and concepts of peer-led 12-step programs.

While living in the TC, every individual participates in communal work managing the facilities and commercial enterprises of the community, providing a matrix of upward mobility and mastery. In some TCs, continuing education and vocational training is highly developed, with members earning college degrees or certified trade expertise.

Progression in the community occurs along three phases of recovery, moving from initial induction to primary treatment to reintegration and planning to leave the community. As re-entry into society nears, issues around post-discharge housing, employment, venues for continued contact with peer-led support groups, and medical and psychiatric follow-up care are addressed to solidify gains made in the community [4, 5, 10].

Purpose of this Book

The frame "Yes, and" structures our discussion of the therapeutic community (TC) model for opioid use disorder (OUD) as we place it within the larger system of care for individuals living with addiction in the United States. Only a minority of patients receive appropriate MAT for OUD, marking a significant treatment gap. Efforts to increase access to these interventions are appropriate and much needed.

And MAT and harm-reduction interventions do not lead to remission or risk reduction for all OUD patients; 6-month retention rates in our best clinical studies of MAT are 30–50% [21]. A significant group continues opioid use with its grave risks despite our first-line treatments. *Yes*, we need to expand access to MAT, *and* we need to diversify the available treatment modalities to reach treatment-resistant populations. Further, MAT and TCs are not exclusive of each other—though there are historical roots to their apparent segregation.

Increased attention to additional treatment approaches for OUD is much needed in the current epidemic. The TC is an effective model that offers a unique treatment frame for treatment-resistant

OUD, yet it is rarely considered an option in the United States and has not been included in the federal response to the opioid crisis.

In this book, the authors explore the historical trends that have shaped the current state of TCs in the American system of care for OUD and other addictions. The opioid epidemic is reviewed alongside our contemporary standard-of-care approaches to OUD. The evidence supporting the TC modality as uniquely effective for treatment-resistant populations are emphasized, including its success in American prisons. Finally, contemporary Italian and Greek models—*San Patrignano* and KETHEA, respectively—are explored in-depth to identify salient mediators of outcome and the unique roles of these TCs in each nation's healthcare system, pointing to the potential place of the TC modality in a diversified response to the opioid epidemic in the United States.

References

1. Clark CD. The recovery revolution: the battle over addiction treatment in the United States. New York: Columbia University Press; 2017.
2. Condelli WS, Hubbard RL. Relationship between time spent in treatment and client outcomes from therapeutic communities. J Subst Abus Treat. 1994;11:25–33.
3. Debaere V, Vanheule S, Inslegers R. Beyond the "black box" of the Therapeutic Community for substance abusers: a participant observation study on the treatment process. Addict Res Theory. 2014;22(3):251–62.
4. DeLeon G. Therapeutic communities. In: Galanter M, Kleber HD, Brady KT, editors. The American psychiatric publishing textbook of substance abuse treatment. 5th ed. Washington, DC: American Psychiatric Publishing; 2015.
5. DeLeon G. "The Gold Standard" and related considerations for a maturing science of substance abuse treatment. Therapeutic Communities; a case in point. Subst Use Misuse. 2015;50(8-9):1106–9.
6. DeLeon G. Is the Therapeutic Community an evidenced based treatment? What the evidence says. Int J Therap Commun. 2010;31(2):104–28.
7. Doogan NJ, Warren K. Semantic networks, schema change, and reincarceration outcomes of therapeutic community graduates. J Subst Abus Treat. 2016;70:7–13.
8. Doherty N, Gottlieb S, McCance-Katz E, Schuchat A, Volkow N. Federal efforts to combat the opioid crisis: a status update on CARA and other initiatives. Testimony to Congressional Senate Committee on Health, Education, Labor & Pensions. Oct 25, 2017. Accessed 1 July 2018 via:

https://www.drugabuse.gov/about-nida/legislative-activities/testimony-to-congress/2017/federal-efforts-to-combat-opioid-crisis-status-update-cara-other-initiatives.
9. Kolodny A, Courtwright DT, Hwang CS, et al. The prescription opioid and heroin crisis: a public health approach to an epidemic of addiction. Annu Rev Public Health. 2015;36:559–74.
10. Kurth DJ. Therapeutic communities. In: Ries RK, Miller SC, Saitz R, Fiellin DA, editors. American Society of Addiction Medicine The ASAM principles of addiction medicine. 5th ed. Philadelphia: Wolters Kluwer Health and Lippincott Williams & Wilkins; 2014.
11. Larochelle MR, Bernson D, Land T, et al. Medication for opioid use disorder after nonfatal opioid overdose and association with mortality. A cohort study. Ann Intern Med . E-publication. 2018;169:137.
12. Ma J, Bao YP, Wang RJ, et al. Effects of medication-assisted treatment on mortality among opioids users: a systematic review and meta-analysis. Mol Psychiatry. 2018.
13. Mattick RP, Breen C, Kimber J, Davoli M. Buprenorphine maintenance versus placebo or methadone maintenance for opioid dependence. Cochrane Database Syst Rev. 2014;2:CD002207.
14. McCance-Katz E, Houry D, Collins F, Gottlieb S. The federal response to the opioid crisis. Testimony to Congressional Senate Committee on Health, Education, Labor & Pensions. Oct 5, 2017. Accessed 1 July 2018 via: https://www.drugabuse.gov/about-nida/legislative-activities/testimony-to-congress/2017/federal-response-to-opioid-crisis.
15. Melnick G, De Leon G, Hiller ML, Knight K. Therapeutic communities: diversity in treatment elements. Subst Use Misuse. 2000;35(12-14):1819–47.
16. National Institute on Drug Abuse. Research reports: Therapeutic Communities: National Institutes of Health; 2015.
17. Sacks S. Overview of therapeutic community outcome research. In: Ries RK, Miller SC, Saitz R, Fiellin DA, editors. American Society of Addiction Medicine The ASAM principles of addiction medicine. 5th ed. Philadelphia: Wolters Kluwer Health and Lippincott Williams & Wilkins; 2014.
18. Substance Abuse and Mental Health Services Administration (SAMHSA). Key substance use and mental health indicators in the United States: Results from the 2017 National survey on drug use and health (HHS Publication No. SMA 18-5068, NSDUH Series H-53). Rockville: Center for Behavioral Health Statistics and Quality, Substance Abuse and Mental Health Services Administration. 2018. Retrieved from https://www.samhsa.gov/data/.
19. Centers for Disease Control and Prevention (CDC). U.S. opioid prescribing rate maps. Oct 3, 2018. Retrieved from https://www.cdc.gov/drugoverdose/maps/rxrate-maps.html.
20. Walley AY, Xuan Z, Hackman HH, et al. Opioid overdose rates and implementation of overdose education and nasal naloxone distribution in Massachusetts: interrupted time series analysis. BMJ. 2013;346:f174. https://doi.org/10.1136/bmj.f174.

21. Williams AR, Nunes EV, Bisaga A, Pincus HA, Johnson KA, Campbell AN, Remien RH, Crystal S, Friedmann PD, Levin FR, Olfson M. Developing an opioid use disorder treatment cascade: a review of quality measures. J Subst Abus Treat. 2018;91:57–68.
22. Sorensen JL, Andrews S, Delucchi KL, et al. Methadone patients in the therapeutic community: a test of equivalency. Drug Alcohol Depend. 2009;100(1-2):100–6.
23. Greenberg B, Hall DH, Sorensen JL. Methadone maintenance therapy in residential therapeutic conmmunity settings: challenges and promise. J Psychoactive Drugs. 2007;39(3):203–10.
24. Dye MH, Roman PM, Knudsen HK, et al. The availability of integrated care in a national sample of therapeutic communities. J Behav Health Ser Res. 2012;39(1):17–27.

Therapeutic Communities: Evolutionary Arc and the Opioid Epidemic

2

George De Leon

Evolutionary Arc

Communities that heal have existed in some form since ancient times. The immediate precursors of the modern addiction therapeutic community (TCs) are readily traced through the genealogy of programs that proliferated during the 1960s and 1970s. Beginning in 1958, TC programs rapidly spawned directly and indirectly from Synanon and Daytop Village. Prominent first-generation programs included, for example, Gateway, Gaudenzia, Integrity House, Marathon House, Odyssey House, Phoenix House, Samaritan Village, Walden House, and Village South. These and other TCs were literally seeded or designed by former members (graduates and dropouts) of a TC directly transmitting common elements of the philosophy, social organization, and practices from their "parent" program ([5]; Chap. 2).

The accelerated diffusion of the TC in North America can be described as a "movement" from the marginal to the mainstream of substance abuse treatment that can be summarized in terms of three major developments: the applications of the approach for special populations and settings, the considerable research

G. De Leon (✉)
Department of Psychiatry, New York University School of Medicine, New York, NY, USA

J. D. Avery, K. A. Kast (eds.), *The Opioid Epidemic and the Therapeutic Community Model*, https://doi.org/10.1007/978-3-030-26273-0_2

documenting the effectiveness and cost benefits of TC treatment, and the emergence of a bona fide TC theory derived from decades of practice and research.

TC Applications

The traditional TC approach is actually the prototype of a variety of TC-oriented programs. Today, the TC modality consists of a wide range of programs serving a diversity of clients who use a variety of drugs and present with complex social and psychological problems in addition to their chemical abuse. Highlighted are some of the key modifications and applications of the TC approach for different patient populations in different settings such as hospitals, shelters, prisons, and day treatment centers.

Most community-based TC agencies have expanded their social services or have incorporated new interventions to address the needs of their diverse residents. These include family services, primary health care specifically geared toward HIV-positive patients and individuals with AIDS [3, 19], aftercare, particularly for substance-abusing inmates leaving prison-based TCs [18], relapse prevention training [17], 12-step groups [3], pharmacotherapy (e.g., psychotropic medications for co-occurring disorders), and mental health services. TCs have also incorporated evidenced-informed psychosocial treatment protocols developed outside of TCs, e.g., cognitive-behavioral therapy, motivational interviewing, and seeking safety. These modifications and additions are intended *to enhance, not substitute for,* community as method, the primary treatment approach.

Many TC agencies are multimodality treatment centers that offer services in their residential and nonresidential settings, depending on the clinical status and situational needs of the individual. These include short-term (less than 90 days), medium-term (6–9 months), and relatively few long-term (1–2 years) residential programs. Attempts are made to match the patient to the appropriate modality within the agency (e.g., short-term residential and ambulatory TC models for more socialized patients). Studies indicate better retention rates for those who are matched to TC-oriented residential and outpatient settings on the basis of multiple domains of drug use severity and social and psychological functioning, compared with those who aren't matched (e.g., [11]).

In its application to special populations, TCs have also adapted the model to comply with the demands of different settings and institutions such as prisons and mental hospitals. In these adapted models the focus on mutual self-help is retained along with the TC recovery perspective. However, issues related to differences in security, regulations, staffing, and philosophy have limited the implementation of the traditional TC program model. An illustrative example of these issues in prison settings is discussed elsewhere (see [9, 14]).

Research

A considerable scientific knowledge base has focused on the effectiveness of the TC (see [7, 20, 22, 24, 25]). The most extensive body of research bearing on the effectiveness of addiction TC programs has amassed from the major national multimodality, multi-year field outcome studies, and notable "case studies" of single community-based TC programs. All of these evaluations employed similar longitudinal designs that collectively followed thousands of admissions to TCs during and up to 5 or more years after leaving treatment.

Findings showed substantial improvements on separate outcome variables (i.e., drug use, criminality, and employment) and on composite indices for measuring individual success. There is a consistent relationship between retention in treatment and positive posttreatment outcomes in TCs. Those who complete treatment show the best outcomes, and among dropouts, length of stay in treatment predicts positive outcomes (see reviews in [7, 22, 25]). Similar findings have been obtained with a smaller number of controlled and comparative studies involving TC programs. And econometric evaluations have found a significant and positive cost-benefit outcome for TC, particularly associated with reduced criminal activity and gains in employment (see [7, 25]).

Research has also provided evidence for the effectiveness of *modified TCs* for special populations (see [4]). These populations include adolescents in various adaptations of the community-based TC [15], inmates in prison-based TCs [18, 27], people with co-occuring substance abuse and psychiatric disorder [21], and addicted mothers and their children [2, 28].

Theory

The TC for addictions emerged a-theoretically, outside of mainstream mental health and social science. Over time a theoretical framework has evolved from clinical practice and research which classifies the TC as unique social learning approach captured in the phrase "community as method" defined as *the purposive use of the community to teach individuals to use the community to change themselves* ([5], Chap. 6).

Although evolved on a trial and error basis, the TC approach contains elements and practices that gain empirical support from abundant behavioral and social psychological research outside of TCs, e.g., peer tutoring (brother–sister mentors), goal attainment (stage-phase program format), behavior modification (consequential privileges and sanctions), and therapeutic alliance (community affiliation). Similarly, social learning *principles* (e.g., role modeling, vicarious learning) are recognizable in mediating individual change in a community context ([5], Chap. 24). Moreover, developing research directly explores TC process utilizing social network methods to study peer interactions (e.g., [16, 26]) and a social identity framework assessing individual recovery (e.g., [1]). These initiatives provide encouraging evidence toward validating key concepts in TC theory.

Evolutionary Issues and Challenges

A defining event in the evolutionary trajectory was the launch of a national organization, Therapeutic Communities of America (TCA) consisting of some 40 member programs who convened an inaugural conference funded by NIDA in January 1976. The published proceedings of that landmark meeting were prescient in capturing the participants' concern with the impact of mainstreaming on the integrity of the approach. As TCs moved into the mainstream, they were committed to treating clients in shorter time and with decreasing resources. They reshaped staffing composition, reduced the planned duration of residential treatment, reset its treatment goals, and, to a considerable extent, altered the approach itself. These changes were framed as threats to the mutual-help identity of the TC [23]. The challenge, then and now, has been to convert threats into opportunities to advance the potential of the TC in the spectrum of human services. Four issues are briefly highlighted that illustrate this challenge: funding, research, workforce, and treatment fidelity.[1]

Funding and Planned Duration of Treatment

The effectiveness of the TC approach has been demonstrated primarily for residential programs with planned durations of treatment of at least 9–12 months. In recent years, however, fiscal support has been steadily decreasing for long-term treatment in general and for residential treatment in particular. Thus, for the large majority of TCs that depend upon public funding, planned duration of treatment has been reduced often *below the threshold* of time needed to yield positive outcomes.

Strategies to cope with these funding pressures must be guided by what is known about the severity of the disorder and the intensity of treatment. Substance abusers with less severe drug use and social and psychological problems can succeed in less intense treatments. However, severe clients such as those in TCs require more intensive ("higher dosage") treatment to succeed.

Short-term residential TC programs cannot achieve the recovery goals of longer-term treatment. If TCs reduce their planned duration of residential treatment to serve clients with severe disorder,

[1]American-influenced TC programs were launched in Europe in the 1960s. Moreover, the success of TCA stimulated development of the World Federation of Therapeutic Communities (WFTC) composed of a number of regional TC organizations worldwide.

they must establish goals that can be *realistically achieved* in a shorter period of time. These goals center on *motivating and preparing clients to continue* in their recovery process beyond their shorter duration in residential treatment.

However, an appropriate "dosage" (threshold) of treatment can be achieved by shortening the duration of residential treatment and *extending* the duration of nonresidential treatment and aftercare. For example, some TC agencies have implemented a long-term protocol using *combinations* of residential and nonresidential settings to *reconstitute* the impact of time in treatment.

A New Research Agenda

Overall, the weight of the research evidence supports the hypothesis that the long-term residential TC is an effective and cost-effective treatment particularly for those with severe drug abuse and social psychological profiles. Given the relatively few randomized, double-blind controlled trials, however, some critics conclude that the effectiveness of the TC has not been "proven."

The relevance of randomized controlled studies for TCs has been discussed elsewhere [7, 8]. This issue aside, new research is needed on the current generation of programs to further document the contribution of the TC as a major health and human services modality including studies that demonstrate (a) *health benefits* (e.g., reduction in drug/alcohol use, social deviancy, increases in employment, education, and overall psychological well-being), (b) *cost benefits* of both long-term TCs and shorter-term residential programs for specific subgroups of substance abusers, and (c) *collateral benefits* (e.g., *prevention* of trans-generational drug use, HIV, STDs, and family breakdown).

Workforce

The expansion of the TC to serve special populations in special settings has resulted in a number of problems in the recruitment, retention, and development of experienced staff. General problems include low salaries, limited career goals, and difficult working conditions. However, a specific workforce issue arises from the *diversity of staff* in TCs. The increased number of traditional professional staff from mental health and social services has posed a special challenge to the TC. Based on their education and training, traditional human services staff utilize concepts, vernacular, and methods that often counter or subvert the fundamental mutual self-help features of the TC. This issue requires strategies that focus on staff integration through didactic and experiential training on the theory and practice of the TC approach (discussed below).

A key integrative element that distinguishes the approach is that regardless of professional background, all staff are *members* of the community and *facilitators* of community as method. These common role features minimize professional differences and underscore that the TC is primarily a *client-driven* treatment approach.

Treatment Fidelity

Understandably, TC organizations have pursued financial solvency by expanding to serve a wide variety of populations, e.g., mental health, homeless, corrections, juvenile justice, and parents with children. Contracts have obligated TCs to meet regulations of community, state, and federal agencies and often to incorporate practices based upon different professional views of treatment. This expansion outward of the TC, however, has been at the expense of *inward* refinement of the approach itself. It is one thing to modify and adapt the TC to special populations, settings, and shorter durations of treatment. It is quite another to ignore the fidelity of the TC's unique approach. TC effectiveness and fidelity of treatment are closely related in that high-fidelity treatment produces better outcomes [13].

Fidelity, meaning "faithful" to the TC approach, may be understood in terms of two dimensions. The first refers to the extent to which programs (a) are guided by the TC perspective on recovery and "right living" for treating the whole person; (b) adhere to its mutual self help approach, community, and method; and (c) retain essential components of the program model (e.g., community meetings, a resident work structure, a phase system, peer encounter, and other groups). The second dimension of fidelity refers to the standards of clinical and management *practice*, i.e., the extent to which the activities and essential components of the program are implemented appropriately and effectively.

To retain its unique identity and effectiveness within mainstream human services, TCs must address the complex issue of treatment fidelity. Training to high fidelity utilizes curricula grounded in TC theory that focuses on 3 related questions: *what, how, and why we do what we do* in therapeutic communities. Moreover, grounding in the TC approach requires *immersion training* formats that provide didactic and experiential learning. These are most efficiently implemented in high-fidelity TC programs that are dedicated *centers of excellence*.[2]

In summary, while the above issues continually challenge the TC, they do not obscure the TC's contributions to drug treatment in the past 50 years. Arguably, the therapeutic community for addictions is the first formal treatment approach that is explicitly *recovery oriented.* Surely, AA and similar mutual self-help approaches facilitate recovery, but these represent themselves as support, not treatment. Pharmacological approaches, notably, methadone and buprenorphine, have as their treatment goal the reduction or elimination of illicit opiate use. Behavioral approaches, such as cognitive behavioral therapy (CBT), contingency contracting, and motivational enhancement (MET), focus upon reduction in targeted drug use behaviors and cognitions. In the TC perspective, however, the primary goal of treatment is

[2]Ironically, the early prototype of such centers appeared in the first generation of community based TCs. Well known programs (e.g. Phoenix House, Daytop Village, Amity) were the sources for developing residents into experienced staff whose expertise evolved from their participation in high fidelity programs. Many of these staff helped to launch new community and prison based programs. Informed by research, formal *didactic* curricula emerged later that articulated theory concepts and rationales. Today, *experiential and didactic* understanding are essential for managing and maintaining high fidelity TCs.

recovery which is broadly defined as changes in lifestyles and identities, along with elimination of substance use/abuse.

Moreover, the research on TCs has documented the *fact* of recovery particularly among serious heroin abusers. Over the years, thousands of individuals have initiated their recovery careers in TC programs. And, though not generally recognized, significant numbers of former TC participants constitute cadres of substance abuse counselors and recovery coaches. In its application to various settings, TCs demonstrated how "community as method" can modify jails, prisons, shelters, hospital wards, or schools to become *change-oriented* environments. The message of change is especially relevant for the disaffiliated in our society and those struggling to acquire a personal and social stake in life. It is a message that is particularly meaningful in the current opioid crisis.

The TC and the Current Opioid Epidemic

Historically, opioid addiction drew little public attention as a *stand alone* health issue to be treated or prevented. Society's response has largely been driven by the *consequences* of addiction. In previous epidemics, for example, overdose death, drug-related crime, drug-use-related HIV, and sexually transmitted diseases (STDs) provided the fuel for igniting public policy to fund treatments for opioid addiction. Currently, the fuel is the alarming rise in overdose deaths, increasingly among all ethnic groups and socioeconomic classes of society.

Actually, the current epidemic of opioid abuse consists of two components, an overuse of prescription drugs (i.e., Oxycontin) and a separate overdose epidemic involving lethal combinations of street drugs, e.g., heroin, fentanyl, and cocaine. Understandably, the public health response to this complex epidemic has focused on strategies to prevent overdose death. These include medication-assisted treatment (MAT) involving methadone or buprenorphine (detox from OxyContin) and Narcan for overdose (over the counter) and needle exchange programs that prevent HIV and HEP C. Though federally prohibited, safe injection facilities, SIFS, are settings where opioids are used without arrests and also provide needle exchange and resuscitation.

The complexity of the present epidemic underscores the need for strategies in addition to MAT and harm reduction. These must address the diversity of people, problems, and social psychological issues associated with drug abuse and the risk of overdose death. Therapeutic communities have demonstrated effectiveness with primary heroin addicts as well as substance abusers for whom effective medications are not available. These include non-opioid abusers, e.g., cocaine/crack, methamphetamine, pill, and polydrug abuse. Untreated, a number of these abusers eventually become heroin involved and at risk for overdose.

Moreover, two models of treatment illustrate the *integration* of the TC and pharmacotherapy for specific subgroups of opiate abusers [6, 10]. Both provide the methadone client with the opportunity for entering the recovery process grounded in a basic assumption; medically assisted treatment can facilitate a recovery process insofar as it eliminates illicit opiate use and retains clients in a treatment setting.

In a methadone to abstinence (M-A) model, clients undergo a gradual detoxification from methadone (usually up to 6 months) while participating in a standard 12-month TC residential program. The effectiveness of M-A programs has not been evaluated in rigorous studies, although long-standing clinical impression has been consistent in reporting positive outcomes for those clients who achieve methadone detoxification and complete their planned residential tenure in the TC.

An intensive day treatment model based on TC methods (passages) has been implemented for methadone-maintained clients who continue to engage in high-risk drug use and sexual behavior [12]. Detoxification from methadone is not essential to recovery. However, abstinence from nonmedically prescribed substances and other risk behaviors is a goal that is achieved by trial-error learning in the recovery process. The efficacy of the passages model has been demonstrated in an open clinical trial at two sites [12]. Though requiring replication, the findings support the larger mission of the project to demonstrate a successful integration of medical-assisted treatment and TC methods for subgroups of methadone-maintained clients.

Beyond the crisis of overdose in the current epidemic, the broader role of therapeutic communities in society's drug problems is illuminated by two related concepts, enculturation and vulnerability. Since the 1960s, epidemics have occurred in an American society in which recreational substance use has become embedded. This *enculturation* of drug use is evident in the following: a continuing increase in the number and type of substances used, both prescribed and non-prescribed, legal and nonlegal, natural and synthetic; the declining age of initial or first use of substances apparent in widespread youth involvement; and the expanded use of substances to all socioeconomic levels, that is, among the advantaged and the disadvantaged. Using a disease analogy, enculturation defines society's chronic involvement with substances while epidemics occur as acute episodes of catastrophic drug abuse.

Enculturation exposes those who are the most *vulnerable* to problematic substance abuse. Genetics, mental and physical health, parental/family relations, and peer influences are some factors that have been implicated in affecting vulnerability. Moreover, social-structural forces, e.g., poverty, economic inequity, and racial/discrimination, have been linked to vulnerability factors in addiction, overall health, and social deviance among significant subgroups in society, the economically disadvantaged, the disaffiliated, and the marginalized. For example, some observers, referring to Appalachia, have characterized the current epidemic as "deaths of despair."[3]

From their inception, therapeutic communities have been serving the most vulnerable substance abusers. For these casualties, medically assisted treatment and harm reduction strategies, while necessary to prevent overdose death, are not sufficient to strengthen their immunity to substance abuse. Epidemics recede, but society's drug problem persists, as does the need for therapeutic communities.

---

[3]Several recent examples are American Fix: Inside the Opioid Addiction Crisis – and How to End It by Ryan Hampton with Clair Rudy Foster. All Points Press. American Overdose: The Opioid Tragedy in Three Acts by Chris McGreal. Public Affairs. Dopesick: Doctors, and the Drug Company That Addicted America by Beth Macy. Little Brown Publisher.

Conclusion

The evolution of TCs reflects the maturation of the addiction treatment field in general. It is some 5 decades since the emergence of an organized field of substance abuse treatment and the mainstreaming of addiction treatment research. The advances are evident in an impressive biomedical, socio-behavioral, genetic, and neuroscience knowledge base. Moreover, the trajectory of treatment policy has moved across perspectives such as chronic disease management, harm reduction, and recently a resurgent recovery movement. The recovery perspective is the fundamental rationale for the TC program model, its unique approach, community as method, and its longer planned duration of treatment. Multidimensional ("whole person") change requires a multi-interventional approach implemented for a sufficient period of time. Thus, in the current opioid epidemic, the TC is reasserting its historical position and mission in the field – that of promoting recovery and right living.

References

1. Beckwith M, Best D, Dingle G, Perryman C, Lubman D. Predictors of flexibility in social identity among people entering a Therapeutic Community for substance abuse. Alcohol Treat Q. 2015;33(1):93–104.
2. Coletti S, Schinka J, Hughes P, Hamilton N, Renard C, Sicilian D, Urman C, Neri R. PAR village for chemically dependent women philosophy and program elements. J Subst Abus Treat. 1995;12(4):289–96.
3. De Leon G. Aftercare in Therapeutic Communities. Int J Addict. 1990–1991;25(9A&10A):1225–37.
4. De Leon G, editor. Community as method: Therapeutic Communities for special populations and special settings. Westport: Greenwood; 1997.
5. De Leon G. The Therapeutic Community; theory, model and method. New York: Springer Publishing; 2000.
6. De Leon G. Integrating maintenance and different therapeutic programming. In: Waal H, Haga E, editors. Maintenance treatment of heroin addiction: evidence at the crossroads. Oslo: J.W. CappelenAkademiskForlag; 2003. p. 296–314.
7. De Leon G. Is the Therapeutic Community an evidence based treatment? What the evidence says. Int J Therap Commun. 2010;31(2):104–75.

8. De Leon G. "The Gold Standard" and related considerations for a maturing science of substance abuse treatment. Therapeutic Communities; a case in point. Subst Use Misuse. 2015;50(8-9):1106–9.
9. De Leon G. In: Ackerman G, Shuker R, editors. Therapeutic Communities for substance abusers in correctional settings: Springer Publications; In Press.
10. De Leon G, Jones HE, Stitzer M. Medication free treatment of opioid dependence. In: Strain EC, Stitzer ML, editors. The treatment of opioid dependence. Baltimore: Johns Hopkins University Press; 2005. p. 323–45.
11. De Leon G, Melnick G, Cleland C. Client matching: a severity-treatment intensity paradigm. J Addict Dis. 2008;27:99–113.
12. De Leon G, Staines GL, Perlis TE, Sacks S, McKendrick K, Hilton R, Brady R. Therapeutic Community methods in methadone maintenance (passages):an open clinical trial. Drug Alcohol Depend. 1995;37(1995):45–57.
13. Dye M, Ducharme L, Johnson J, Knudsen H, Roman P. Modified Therapeutic Communities and adherence to traditional elements. J Psychoactive Drugs. 2009;41(3):275–83.
14. Hiller ML, Saum CA. Substance abuse treatment in prison: the Therapeutic Community. In: Church WT, Springer D, editors. Serving the stigmatized: working within the incarcerated environment. New York: Oxford University Press; 2018.
15. Jainchill N. Therapeutic Communities for adolescents; the same and not the same. In: Community as method: Therapeutic Communities for special populations and special settings. Westport: Greenwood; 1997.
16. Kreager DA, Bouchard M, De Leon G, Schaeffer DR, Soyer M, Young JT, Zajac G. A life course and networks approach to prison Therapeutic Communities. In: Social networks in the life course. Cham: Springer; 2018. p. 433–51.
17. Lewis B, Ross R. Retention in Therapeutic Communities: challenges for the nineties HIV: advances in research and applications. NIDA Research Monograph Series no. 144 1994, 232-25899=116; 1994.
18. Martin S, Butzin CA, Saum CA, Inciardi JA. Three year outcomes of Therapeutic Community treatment for drug involved offenders in Delaware. Prison J. 1999;79(3):291–320.
19. McCusker J, Sorensen J. HIV and Therapeutic Communities in Therapeutic Community: advances in research and applications. NIDA Research Monograph Series no. 144; 1994, pp. 232–258.
20. National Institute On Drug Abuse Research Report Series; Therapeutic Community. What is a Therapeutic Community?. Rockville: National Institute on Drug Abuse; 2002, 2015.
21. Sacks S, Banks S, McKendrick K, Sacks J. Modified Therapeutic Community for co-occurring disorders: a summary of four studies. J Subst Abus Treat. 2008;34(1):112–22.

22. Simpson DD, Curry SJ, editors. Drug abuse treatment outcome studies (DATOS). Psychol Addict Behav. 1997;11(special issue 4):211–337.
23. The Therapeutic Community. Proceedings of Therapeutic Communities of America planning conference, Jan. 29–30, 1976. DHEW Publication No.(ADM) 77-464.
24. Tims F, De Leon G, Jainchill N, editors. 1994 Advances in research and applications. NIDA Research Monograph Series no. 144, 1994.
25. Vanderplasschen W, Colbert K, Autrique M, Rapp RC, Peace S, Broekaert E, Vandevelde S. Therapeutic Communities for addictions: a review of their effectiveness from a recovery-oriented perspective. Sci World J. 2013;2013:1–22.
26. Warren KL, Doogan N, De Leon G, Phillips GS, Moody J, Hodge A. Short-run prosocial behavior in response to receiving corrections and affirmations in three Therapeutic Communities. J Offender Rehabil. 2013;52(4):270–86.
27. Wexler HK, Prendergast ML. Therapeutic Communities in United States' prisons: effectiveness and challenges. Ther Communities. 2010;31:157–75.
28. Winick C, Evans J. A Therapeutic Community Program for mothers and their children. In: De Leon G, editor. Community as method: Therapeutic Communities for special populations and special settings. Westport: Greenwood; 1997.

The Modern Therapeutic Community Model

3

Fernando B. Perfas

Introduction

The TC has been around for six decades and continues to be the treatment of choice for government and nongovernment drug treatment programs in the USA and in different parts of the world. In the course of its dispersion, as it was adopted in different cultural settings, changes have been made to adapt its practice to local realities as well as suit the preferences of various professionals. Some of the changes have diverged from the original TC concept which resulted to inconsistent and bad practices. When the TC first rose into prominence as a promising treatment approach to narcotics addiction of the 1960s, the political and social environment was very different from where we find ourselves today. Its relevance in the face of the changing drug abuse and drug treatment landscapes is sometimes questioned. The why and how it worked has always been the subject of debates. It wasn't until the 1980s that results of outcome studies of its effectiveness started to come out [1, 2, 4, 14]. The first book that described the TC model, its theory and methods, came out only in 2000 when De Leon [10] published his book on the TC for addictions. During its time as the popular treatment model for addiction, not much has been written about its treatment philosophy and methods. The mode of instruction was

F. B. Perfas (✉)
Addiction Training Consultant, Red Hook, NY, USA

J. D. Avery, K. A. Kast (eds.), *The Opioid Epidemic and the Therapeutic Community Model*, https://doi.org/10.1007/978-3-030-26273-0_3

largely experiential through actual treatment. For most of the 1960s through the 1980s, the workforce in TCs across America consisted mostly of ex-addicts who went through TC treatment and who decided to become TC staff. Scholarly tradition grounded on critical analysis and probing the rationale behind the TC rituals, treatment tools, and prevailing practices was not part of the TC culture. In the long run, the entrenched anti-intellectual and anti-professional attitude of some of the early TC leaders did not serve the TC well.

There is limited literature that provides helpful practice guidelines or standard practice of how the various TC tools should be implemented. Much less are the literature expounding on theories that explain why such tools work. Despite these limitations the TC has proven resilient and relevant as a treatment model. A TC can be defined as a recovery-oriented drug-free treatment environment for people with addiction who live in an organized and structured community to achieve personal change through self-help and mutual help process.

A Brief Retrospective Look at Therapeutic Community for Addictions in America

The TC for addictions, otherwise known as the *concept-based or hierarchical therapeutic community,* traces its origin to the Synanon model that was started by an ex-alcoholic, Charles Dederich, and his cohorts in 1958 [30]. In contrast, the TC that developed a decade earlier in Great Britain, which was largely pioneered by British psychiatrists and designed to treat mental illness, was known as the *democratic therapeutic community* [25]. Since its rise to fame and eventual fall, when Dederich turned Synanon into a cultish movement, the addiction treatment model that he started had been replicated in different parts of North America and eventually the rest of the world. In the height of its popularity, Dederich made an important ideological change in the direction of the Synanon program. He declared Synanon a closed TC where membership was for life and the goal of treatment was not anymore the eventual reintegration of members back to society [13]. This resulted to other TCs that believed social reintegration to be the ultimate goal of drug treatment to part ways with Synanon.

When the TC first emerged in the addiction treatment scene of the late 1950s, the USA was in the throes of a serious heroin epidemic. Without any viable treatment for narcotic addiction at the time, an addict was often viewed as suffering from a terminal condition. "Once an addict, always an addict," was the mantra for many decades. The TC model as expounded by Synanon showed promise, a breakthrough in the often bleak treatment landscape of addiction. Hopes were high as increasing ex-addict members, many of whom were ex-convicts, were not only able to remain drug-free but were able to hold responsible roles in the Synanon organization.

Before long TC programs spread to big cities of the USA and Canada. Thanks to several ex-Synanon members who helped start many of these drug programs. Together with the growth of the TC was the rise of a new profession, the birth of the *ex-addict paraprofessionals* [7]. They were to become the unchallenged authority in the implementation and practice of the TC in several of these treatment institutions. For many years only TC "graduates" were entitled to the imminent position of a TC director. This was a very unique feature in the staffing pattern of the traditional TC. This practice lasted until recently as more academically trained addiction and medical personnel are being required to operate licensed drug treatment programs. The change coincided with the decline in funding for nonprofit TCs from the federal and state governments and increased emphasis on professionalizing the addiction workforce through various state addiction credentialing certification boards.

By the late 1980s and mid-1990s, the shift in the TC staffing pattern was evident, with increasing numbers of professionals joining the ranks of TC staff, most of whom had backgrounds in social work, psychology, and medical or mental health fields [23]. This trend was bolstered by the growth in the addiction treatment industry and enabled by the inclusion of accredited college courses toward certifications as addiction counselors. Overnight, the TC saw the influx of inexperienced albeit certified addiction counselors working side by side with ex-addict TC graduate staff. They were hired mostly to meet funding regulations that required certified professional addiction workforce. Meanwhile, many of the TC veteran ex-addict paraprofessionals were aging, and the lack of a thoughtfully designed training program to train nonaddict professional staff in the art and science of TC work was severely lacking. These and other factors, such as the increased efforts by state regulatory boards to curtail traditional TC practices and the diminished funding stream, have contributed to the decline of many large therapeutic communities that were established during the height of the TC movement in the USA.

When cocaine and crack superseded heroin or opiates as the leading drugs of abuse in the USA in the 1980s, there were questions in the minds of some experts as to the TC's relevance as a treatment approach for non-narcotic drug users. About this time also, the results of the landmark outcome study on the effectiveness of the TC [9] were getting a lot of attention. Several succeeding large replication studies produced and confirmed previous findings. Additionally, the thriving in-prison therapeutic communities were also coming out with their own impressive outcome studies that further confirmed the effectiveness of TC even in a nonvoluntary treatment setting. By this time the average length of treatment in many TCs had been reduced to a year due to a drastic reduction of government funding. At the same time criminal justice agencies that contracted TCs for drug treatment services negotiated shorter-term treatment for their clients. By the 1990s the overwhelming majority of client populations in large nonprofit TCs such as Daytop Village, Phoenix House, Odyssey House, or Samaritan Village were from the criminal justice system, e.g., drug courts, parole and probation, etc. In some cases, these TCs operated drug programs within the prison. The demographics of client populations up to this time in most nonprofit TCs have remained relatively stable, with large proportions of African Americans and Hispanics from urban areas. This, however, was about to change.

In the aftermath of the cocaine/crack epidemic, we saw the dramatic increase in the number of substance abuse disorder (SUD) clients in TCs with co-occurring psychiatric conditions. Not long after, research on psychological trauma or post-traumatic stress disorder (PTSD) began to pour in, establishing the highly significant relationships between trauma and SUD with the majority of clients in treatment having had one form of serious psychological trauma or another [20]. These developments caught the TC unprepared to deal with the large majority of clients that require psychiatric interventions and monitoring. This has resulted in a serious departure from a cornerstone traditional TC treatment philosophy: drug-free treatment. The increasing numbers of clients with co-occurring disorders have to be put on psychiatric medications as part of treatment [24]. New methods of managing these clients in TC and a readjustment of staffing patterns that require more professionals with mental health backgrounds were needed. New organizational model that combines a business approach and incorporates trauma-informed treatment approaches was sorely needed.

By the turn of the century, a gradual shift begun to occur in the demographics of the TC treatment populations, particularly in the US East Coast-based TCs. By the early 2000s there was an influx of criminal justice drug offenders coming from small cities and towns in the rural areas of the country with large Caucasian populations. The opioid epidemic was now in full swing fueled by narcotic pharmaceuticals and the flow into the USA of cheaper narcotic called fentanyl and South American heroin. The drug trend in the USA had come full circle with pharmaceutical opioids on the rise and heroin making a comeback, albeit with a different SUD clients' demographics, which was largely represented not by the usual urban poor and minorities but by a largely white working class and young-adult populations.

Ironically, while the opioid epidemic was raging, the traditional large TCs were going through financial difficulties and under increasing scrutiny because of some TC practices taken out of context and viewed as antiquated. The traditional large TCs struggled to adopt a business model to make operations financially viable. Meanwhile, funding agencies and health insurance companies were reluctant to finance a longer-term treatment and favored shorter behavioral health approaches. This political and economic environment and the inability to adapt to the shifting realities of drug treatment contributed to the decline of the large traditional TCs.

The Leadership in TC

The leadership style practiced in Synanon was autocratic and patriarchal with Charles Dederich, who sat on top of the Synanon hierarchical totem pole, as the final arbiter of debates on major policy [3, 30]. It wasn't unusual that he made unilateral decisions on controversial organizational policies. Within a tight-knit community, a strong sense of family led by a charismatic father figure was attractive to many who suffered from lifelong feelings of alienation and rejection. Synanon and the TCs that came after, which were referred to as first-generation TCs, all seem to have adopted the leadership culture of Synanon. Although most of these TCs were governed by a board of trustees, the founding leader or leaders often sat as president, chairman, or chief executive officer and each opinion held sway in the organization. Under this climate, only select individuals, usually ex-addict TC graduate who earned the trust of the leadership, were able to make important organizational decisions or policy changes. The leadership was considered the sole authority and expert on the TC model.

This leadership style and the TC moralistic stance, which are Synanon legacies, did not encourage initiative from the TC workforce to engage in critical discussions of the TC methods for fear of contradicting the official line handed down from the top. Embracing a line of thinking that differed from the official interpretation of the TC was considered rouge. This could also cause one to get ostracized from the organization. This led to the anti-intellectual climate of the early TCs and its conservative intellectual culture. This, however, was the step taken to protect the TC from becoming corrupted or at least a particular interpretation of the TC from being revised.

The Theoretical Framework of the TC

The application of theories that underlie the practice of the TC is more of an afterthought rather than a deliberate process. The developers and practitioners of early TCs did not set out to construct theoretical models about human behavior and then apply and test them through research. The originators of the addiction TC were pragmatists, not academicians, with good intuitive grasp of human behavior involved in addiction. Although Dederich showed deep interest in Eastern thoughts, the writings of Emerson, and used sprinklings of psychoanalytic and behaviorist ideas to elaborate on Synanon approaches [30], early TC practitioners, for the most part, did not care to look for formal theories that could explain, for example, how people change. It became the task of later writers to sort out theories that can explain the how and why TC work. One important insight that was evident was their understanding of the power of the group, the community, to have far-reaching influences on a member's behavior.

Modern TC's theoretical base can be described as eclectic, a sort of a trans-theoretical model that includes psychoanalytic, behavior and cognitive-behavioral, humanistic, existential, and social learning theories, among others. For example, Deitch [8], an ex-Synanon member and a TC pioneer who brought the TC concept to Daytop Village in 1963, conceptualized the TC treatment tools and group processes in largely behaviorist and psychoanalytic terms. This makes sense for a treatment model that is more concerned with practice rather than develop theories that explain why its practices work. The TC is not beholden to any school of thought or a particular theoretical orientation.

Diffusion and Evolution of Modern Therapeutic Communities: Issues and Concerns

It is estimated that there are 3000 therapeutic communities globally in community-based programs, hospitals, prisons, juvenile centers, orphanages, government treatment centers, etc. It remains the choice treatment model for various drug rehabilitation programs that serve different classes of drug users and drug offenders [11].

In the course of time as the TC was adopted and adapted in different settings and cultures, it had undergone transformations in both form and substance. *Form* refers to how TC practices are implemented, for example, the behavior-shaping tools, morning meeting, learning experience, etc., and how the rituals that come with them are put to use. *Substance* pertains to the real intent or underlying rationale for the TC practices that are consistent with the TC philosophy. For example, the *learning experience (LE)* in the TC is meant to teach, not punish, although in appearance the learning task being asked of the person on an LE has the element of a punishment. People who are removed from the actual process of how an LE is set up, which is designed according to the nature of the offense and the learning goal for the individual, can readily see it as a form of punishment. This misunderstanding accounts for the egregious abuses of clients in some TCs in the name of the learning experience. The substance of the TC or its philosophical foundation is what makes it a distinct treatment approach. When this is lost, the practice of the TC will consist of nothing but empty rituals. The form of the TC can vary due to different factors such as the type of setting or cultural realities, but its substance must remain intact if we are to guarantee its fidelity.

The behavior-shaping tools, such as the "verbal haircut" or reprimand, "pull-up," etc., are another source of controversy because of their apparent harshness and clash with some cultural norms, especially in cultures that shun the display of strong emotions. What is often missed is the spirit of *responsible concern* that underlies the practice of these tools. Part of the process in the practice of these tools is a thoughtful review of who should be involved, what behavioral issue has to be addressed, and how the intervention should be delivered. The recipient must feel that it is all about him and his transgression, and the intervention is an honest effort to help him despite the bluntness of how it is put to him. Often people focus on the form of the intervention, not its substance. Furthermore, it is not uncommon for drug programs that adopt the TC to have the mistaken notion that the TC is largely a set of behavior-shaping interventions and that is all. What they don't understand is that the behavior-shaping tools are means of threshing and winnowing the course behavior and attitude that accompany addictive behavior. Their practice is meant to psychologically prime the person for the harder and more demanding process of emotional and cognitive change.

An important philosophical feature of the TC that is simple enough to wrap our head around is *community as method*, and yet when putting it to practice, we see all sorts of problems and inconsistencies. De Leon [11] defines community as method as "the purposive use of the community to teach individuals to utilize the community to change themselves." There is an important TC concept that provides an important link to it. The TC must be a *peer-driven process* to lend itself to *community as method.* Without sufficient experience and understanding of how the TC actually works, the nuances in the practice of these concepts are easy to miss. The TC treatment process largely involves various forms of peer interactions from the practice of the behavior-shaping tools to probing and providing emotional support to each other in groups and other activities. The TC members are organized in a social hierarchy of peers who move up the organizational ladder based on their ability to live up to the TC norms, values, and community behavioral standards. This social hierarchy is also referred to as the *structure* which is the most important means of empowering TC members and which helps them achieve emotional and social maturity as the TC replicates society at large, although in a more controlled environment. Members of staff who are also integral part of the community lead from behind and only intervene when necessary. Perhaps the substance of this aspect of the TC is often missed when adopting and adapting the TC in different settings. Figure 3.1 provides a graphic representation of how *community as method* is operationalized in a typical TC [22].

Additionally, the TC can be conceptualized as *bimodal* comprised of a *social system* and a *therapeutic model* [22]. As a social system the TC provides the organizing principles of how and when treatment or interventions are implemented, thereby creating a context that is conducive for therapeutic processes to occur. As a treatment model, it is comprised of overlapping but distinct behavioral, psychological, social, moral, and cognitive strategies or approaches designed to achieve positive change in addictive behaviors. The social system and clinical approaches overlap and are reciprocal so that the integrity of the system is dependent on the proper practice of the TC tools or interventions. The proper implementation of the TC tools is responsible for creating the

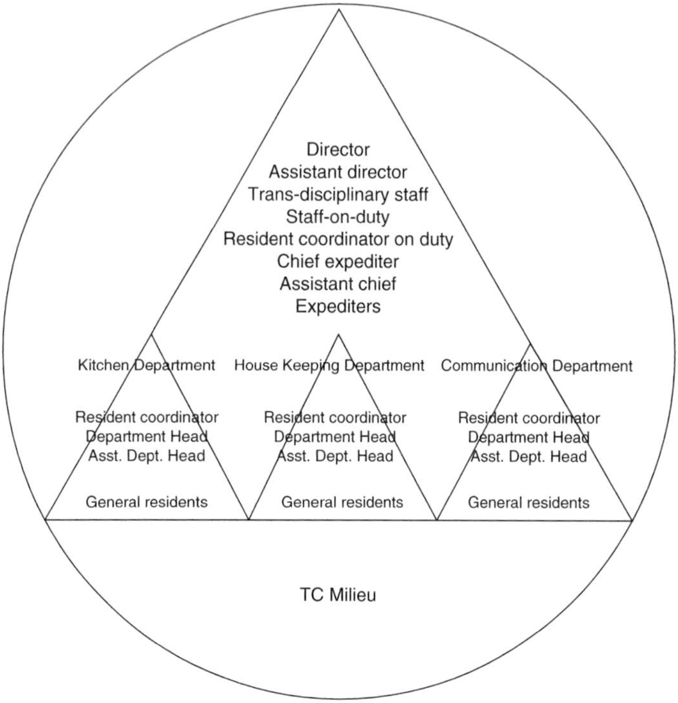

Fig. 3.1 Components of the TC hierarchical social structure

necessary context for change to occur. "Two sides of the same coin" is an apt metaphor for this. This conceptualization of the TC helps one understand how the TC works.

The Structural Components and Practice Principles of the TC*

The TC can be conceptualized using social systems perspective. In this model there are five structural components of the TC, namely, treatment structure, treatment condition, staff role and function, biopsychosocial interventions, and treatment outcome and feedback. Under each component are the practice principles. The components that are outlined below are the *structures* which feature the underlying order that guides the operational performance of the TC. The practice principles are *functions* representing the actual TC performance and activities. These principles can be considered the necessary ingredients of a TC as the application of these principles helps create a context where therapy can occur [22].

1. Treatment Structure

Treatment structure pertains to the social organization of the TC and how treatment activities are organized and implemented. These are outlined in the following principles:

- Principle 1. *There is a progression of treatment through outlined phases.*
- Principle 2. *There is a process for joining the community that explores treatment motivation and promotes belongingness.*
- Principle 3. *There is an orientation process that educates, engages, and facilitates the integration of new residents into the community.*
- Principle 4. *There is a process for separating from the community.*
- Principle 5. *Community members are organized into a social hierarchy with a structure of responsibilities.*

*Detailed discussions on this topic can be found in Perfas F. Therapeutic community: Past, present, and moving forward. New York: Hexagram Publishing; 2014.

2. Treatment Condition

Treatment condition refers to the requirements necessary to establish a safe and adequate TC environment. This is accomplished by practicing the following principles:

- Principle 1. *Safety is foremost.*
- Principle 2. *The treatment process must be dynamic and pervasive.*

- Principle 3. *The TC is a peer-driven treatment process that emphasizes personal responsibility.*
- Principle 4. *The treatment process promotes a culture of self-help and mutual help.*
- Principle 5. *There are shared community norms and values that guide residents' personal conduct.*

3. Staff Role and Function

This component provides the guidelines on how staff should contribute to the formation of the TC environment and maintenance of its operations. It describes unique staff role and functions in the TC.

- Principle 1. *The staffing pattern follows a transdisciplinary model.*
- Principle 2. *The staff members carry out their roles and responsibilities as role models and rational authority.*
- Principle 3. *To operationalize the concept of "community as method," staff must function at three levels of operations: the community level, the individual resident level, and the level of feelings and emotions.*
- Principle 4. *There is a system for training and supervising the different levels of residents' social hierarchy.*

4. Biopsychosocial Treatment Interventions

This component describes the overlapping but distinct categories of TC interventions that include the behavior-shaping tools, reward system and motivational incentives, psychological interventions, medical and psychiatric services, intellectual and moral development, vocational and survival skills development, preparations for social reintegration, and family program.

- Principle 1. *There is a set of behavior-shaping strategies and a system of sanctions on "deviant behaviors."*
- Principle 2. *There is a structured reward system of privileges and motivational incentives.*

- *Principle 3. Medical and mental health services are available to assess, intervene, and monitor medical and psychiatric conditions that co-occur with substance abuse.*
- Principle 4. *Community members are provided with interventions and activities that help resolve psychological problems and promote emotional growth.*
- Principle 5. *The community provides interventions and activities that enhance intellectual abilities, self-awareness, moral reasoning, and self-actualization.*
- Principle 6. *The community provides interventions and activities that increase personal competency and survival skills.*
- Principle 7. *The community provides interventions and activities that promote pro-social values and social reintegration.*
- Principle 8. *The TC includes a family program that engages and provides support for families and significant others.*

5. Treatment Outcome and Feedback

This component refers to gathering feedback through research and program evaluation to determine TC performance and accomplishment of its goals.

- Principle 1. *There is a system for monitoring and evaluating the effectiveness of the therapeutic community and its treatment outcomes.*

Hybridization of the Therapeutic Community

A standard practice regarding how the various TC tools are to be implemented is badly needed. There has never been a "how to" guideline or a standard operational manual available for practicing the TC interventions. Melnick and De Leon [17] created the *Therapeutic Community Essential Elements Scale Questionnaire* (SEEQ) which provided a good template for creating a practice manual. However, the SEEQ is being used mostly in evaluating TC programs. The British *Community of Communities* [5] under the Royal College of Psychiatrists has also published its own *Service Standards for Therapeutic Communities*. A version of it can be found in *Deconstructing the Therapeutic Community* [21]. Although it identifies important elements that must be included in organizing a TC, it does not provide clear guidelines on how the TC tools should be practiced. How much the TC has drifted away from the original concept can be attributed to the absence of a clear standard for implementing the TC tools. In the course of its cultural diffusion throughout the world, it had been molded and remolded and fused with other treatment models. I call this process the *hybridization* of the TC which describes the evolution and transformation of the TC as it has been adopted in different settings [22]. This resulted in the proliferations of TCs across the globe with limited or lack of fidelity to TC practice. The concept was an adaptation of paleoanthropologist Chris Stringer's [26] when he described hybridization as the network of pattern created by gene flow between evolutionarily separate lineages. Hybridization is the result of interbreeding of ancient species of human forebears. It is an analogy describing the outcome of the marriage between the TC and other ideologies.

The hybridization process takes different forms. It is influenced by personal ideologies or professional training or by the leadership responsible for adopting the TC. Cultural and societal beliefs about addiction or the institutional mission of the host organization dictate what features of the TC are installed and what are discarded or revised. The political and treatment infrastructure of the host country, such as the national drug control policy, determines the level of sophistication and the treatment approach to addiction. All these factors contribute to how treatment organizations adopt and adapt the TC. Figure 3.2 depicts the hybridization of the TC through cultural diffusion [22].

One of the consequences of hybridization is "cultural drift," to borrow Stringer's [26] words, a moving away from the original TC concept and philosophical approach. Some of the changes to the TC are not intentional but rather the result of misunderstanding the original concept or its underlying philosophy. Changes are often made to meet requirements or harmonize the TC with the prevailing cultural norms of the new setting. When the revision

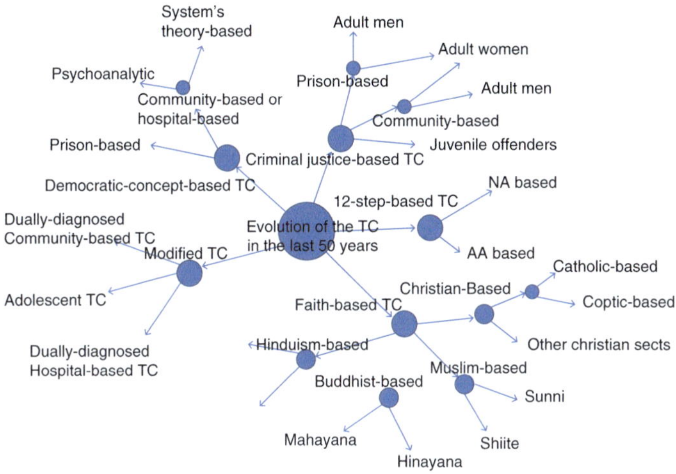

Fig. 3.2 Hybridization of the TC through cultural diffusion

only concerns the form or the ritualistic aspect of the TC and leaves the underlying TC philosophy intact, the fidelity of the TC is kept. Some changes involve tweaking some practices or the addition of new elements to the TC as new knowledge on addiction and the treatment of addiction become available. These new information often come from research or field experience and form the "best practices" of drug treatment. This form of revision when thoughtfully implemented enhances the effectiveness of the TC and does not undermine its fidelity. An example is the inclusion of motivational incentives to complement the TC privileges. While the TC privileges are earned based on time spent in TC and meritorious behavior, motivational incentives reward target behavior regardless of time in the TC program [21]. Keeping fidelity in mind, the TC is flexible enough to accommodate evidence-based practices. The key is to view the TC as a treatment platform, a social system that has its own requirements for optimum functioning.

Toward a Trauma-Informed Therapeutic Community

The landmark study called *Adverse Childhood Experiences* (ACE) [12] and several other studies [16, 29] have presented incontrovertible evidence of the significant relationships between psychological trauma, in the form of early childhood adversity or PTSD, and substance abuse. Furthermore, battered women who are treated for SUD, including children who are witnesses to the abuse, have presented symptoms of PTSD. In fact, several studies have shown that a large number of SUD clients in drug treatment have histories of adverse life experience or trauma [18, 19, 27]. Often the underlying trauma presents itself as other forms of co-occurring disorders such as depression, anxiety, bipolar disorder, personality disorder, etc. [28]. This situation complicates the treatment and management of SUD clients with serious trauma background. They do not respond well to traditional treatment approaches and often fail to complete drug treatment. Their clinical presentation baffles drug treatment counselors who are unfamiliar with psychological trauma. They present more complex problems that go beyond the usual conceptualization of an SUD client. Their drug use is driven by the need to cope with trauma symptoms rather than the desire for the drug high [15]. The deep-seated fear and mistrust that arise from their trauma history present serious challenges in establishing therapeutic relationship and the feeling of safety in the treatment environment.

The "old school" TC approach which is highly intrusive and directive is at odds with the treatment needs of SUD clients with trauma. The pressing agenda for the TC is to take a second look at its tools and interventions, treatment goals, staffing pattern and training, and how clients are managed within the TC. It has to reevaluate its treatment approaches with a trauma lens if it were to remain relevant in the prevailing drug treatment environment. From humanistic, social learning, and cognitive-behavioral perspectives, the TC concept and philosophy offer important elements that are rational and highly humanizing and socializing. Recovery from addiction and trauma should occur within a social context [6]. To break out from the stifling shell of isolation and alienation brought about by trauma experiences and addiction, clients must be able to reexamine old relationships and learn to forge new ones that are safe and healthy. The TC's emphasis on the spirit of community could help facilitate this process.

Clinical Supervision

TCs, at least the traditional TC, eschewed the practice of clinical supervision. The perception was that it is too academic sounding and highly associated with the medical and mental health treatment model which the TC is not. The authoritarian leadership style of the early TCs was not conducive for clinical supervision to flourish since the upper leadership echelon was the only authority on the TC. However, for the modern TCs the practice of clinical supervision would be an example of an adoption of best practice that has several advantages.

Staff burnout is common among addiction workers. The type of clients and the nature of work with SUD all contribute to creating a physically and emotionally demanding job with an already stressful work environment. Moreover, it is not uncommon that those attracted to the often thankless work of drug treatment and rehabilitation are themselves dealing with their own unresolved psychological wounds. Their attraction to addiction work may be a desperate and an unconscious attempt to vicariously heal themselves as they try to "help" others. The TC is a highly emotionally charged environment due to various therapeutic processes that are constantly taking place. Staff with unresolved personal issues are vulnerable to adverse or inadequate form of coping. This can manifest in poor judgment or inappropriate behavior and relationship. This puts into perspective the absolute need for clinical supervision to be incorporated into the TC work culture. The combination of personal vulnerabilities and work-related stress puts staff at risk for poor decision-making and burnout. Lastly, the use of clinical supervision is integral to making the TC a trauma-informed treatment.

Why the TC Works

Cozolino [6] describes psychotherapy as a relationship-based learning environment grounded in the history of our social brains, with roots going back to mother-child bonding, attachment to family and friends, and the guidance of wise elders. The description is based on his argument that at the root of what ails most humans who seek therapy is a failure in relationship. This is an allusion to the primal importance of the infant and mother (or caregiver) adequate bonds as determinant in shaping the infant's social brain and his future social adaptation. Our health, more specifically, mental health, is determined prior to and after birth by environmental forces that shape early brain development. How the brain is shaped plays a fundamental role in how the mind is shaped. The mind, on the other hand, is capable of altering the brain via conscious changes in thoughts, actions, and emotions. "The brain is a social organ of adaptation shaped by evolution to connect with and change through interactions with others." Treatment or therapy is harnessing the ability of our brains to link with, synch, and learn from one another to achieve adaptive change. This interaction between the ability among people to connect and learn from one another has been shaped through millennia of social evolution.

For Cozolino, recovery from dysfunctions that arise from difficulties in self-regulation, such as trauma or addictive disorders, must occur in a social context. To paraphrase his description of psychotherapy vis a vis the TC, the TC can be described as a relationship-based structured social learning environment grounded in the social nature of addictive disorders; it is a community composed of members who engage in a healing process through self-help and mutual help.

From an attachment theory perspective, the TC works based on an important principle that "exposure to people changes people." Powerful attachment experiences can alter a person's nervous system, and salient emotionally charged experiences can potentially alter how his brain is wired. In a TC where members have opportunities to establish attachment relationships, they learn to regulate their nervous system and acquire implicit knowledge of the rules involved in healthy relationships [22].

Like other forms of psychotherapy, the TC works because it harnesses our fundamental nature as social beings. The added advantage is that more than the one-to-one social dynamic that occurs in psychotherapy, a TC member is exposed to a mosaic of relationships with peers. The same peers bring to treatment a variety of life issues which provide different perspectives to a person's own difficulties. The sense of community the TC provides is a safe haven where the person can develop multiple attachment figures based on mutual concern. This affords him opportunities to explore and work through intense feelings of anger, hostilities, ambivalence, etc., related to his failures in relationships. He can be confident that he can rise above these otherwise overpowering emotions.

The social context is the "community" where members find solace in the company of others like him. The group provides moderating influences on negative feelings associated with failure to repair oneself by resorting to substance abuse. Various forms of groups and meetings afford members the setting to explore and disentangle difficult emotions related to past relationships in multiple types and levels of transferences within the safety of the community.

Conclusion

Pressures from the changing treatment climate have forced the TC to be flexible in its approaches with increasing focus on client differences, a TC treatment that fits to the needs of the individual and not vice versa. Individualized treatment planning and case management have to be included in the TC practices to make it responsive to the changing client population with trauma or co-occurring disorder. Working in a TC requires staff to engage in regular emotional processing to sharpen their awareness of personal feelings that are triggered by various therapeutic processes. Individual and group supervision will be the ideal setting for accomplishing this.

The TC treatment has proven effective among SUD clients who abuse a variety of substances. It continues to remain a relevant treatment model up to now. Besides its highly structured treatment environment, a fully functioning TC offers comprehensive biopsychosocial approaches that address the behavioral, psychological, cognitive, moral, social, vocational, and medical needs of SUD clients.

Learning the TC happens in two levels: cognitively and experientially. The most common mistake in practicing the TC can be attributed to poor staff training. Learning the TC requires a cognitive understanding of its concepts, theories, and principles that support its treatment tools and its major structural components that include distinct and overlapping treatment interventions. Equally important is grasping experientially how all these come together when implementing the TC.

A good start for the TC to become truly a trauma-informed treatment is to include screening and assessment protocols for psychological trauma as part of client admission, provide training on trauma for staff, and make clinical supervision a standard practice. It also must include trauma in treatment planning and case management. Finally, the TC must examine its interventions with a trauma lens.

Emphasis on community as the healing environment for the stigmatizing and alienating social maladies like addiction is the key to the TC's continued success. Addiction and its underlying causes are better addressed in a social context, and the TC provides a rich and dynamic sociopsychological environment that helps members explore new and different ways of coping.

References

1. Bale RN, Van Stone WW, Kuldau JM, et al. Therapeutic communities versus methadone maintenance: a prospective controlled study of narcotic addiction treatment: design and one-year follow-up. Arch Gen Psychiatry. 1980;37(2):179–93.
2. Bale RN, Zarcone VP, Van Stone WW, Kuldau JM, et al. Three therapeutic communities. A prospective controlled study of narcotic addiction

treatment: process and two-year follow-up results. Arch Gen Psychiatry. 1984;41(2):185–91.
3. Casriel D. The story of Synanon. Beverly Hills: Book Company of America (Printice- Hall, Inc.); 1963.
4. Coombs RH. Back on the streets: Therapeutic communities' impact upon drug users. Am J Drug Alcohol Abuse. 1981;8(2):185–201.
5. Community of Communities. The service standards for Therapeutic Communities. 5th ed: The Royal College of Psychiatrists; 2006.
6. Cozolino L. Why therapy works: using our mind to change. New York: W.W. Norton & Company; 2016.
7. Deitch DA. The end of the beginning: dilemmas of the paraprofessional in current drug abuse treatment. In: Senay E, Alksne H, editors. Developments in the field of drug abuse: proceedings of the national drug abuse conference. Cambridge, MA: Schenkman; 1974. p. 1029–36.
8. Deitch D. The therapeutic community trainer's guide. New York: Daytop International; 1992.
9. De Leon G. The therapeutic community: study of effectiveness. National Institute on Drug Abuse Treatment Research Monograph Series (ADM 84-1286). Washington, DC: Superintendent of Documents, U.S. Government Printing Office; 1984.
10. De Leon G. Therapeutic community: theory, model, and method. New York: Springer Publishing Company; 2000.
11. De Leon G. Modern therapeutic community for addiction. The Quest for right living in modern TCs. https://www.thefix.com/content/therapeutic-communities-George-De-Leon-professional-voices0514, 2015.
12. Felitti V. The origin of addiction: evidence from the Adverse Childhood Experiences Study. Kindheitserfahrungen," Praxis der Kinderpsychologie und Kinderpsychiatrie, 2003;52:547–59. https://attachmentdisorderhealing.com/resources/key-articles/.
13. Gerstel D. Paradise incorporated: Synanon. Novato: Presidio Press; 1982.
14. Holland S. Evaluating community-based treatment programs: a model for strengthening inferences about effectiveness. Int J Therap Commun. 1983;4(4):285–306.
15. Mate G. In the realm of hungry ghosts. Berkeley: North Atlantic Books; 2010.
16. Mate G. Addiction: childhood trauma, stress, and the biology of addiction. J Restorative Med. 2012;1:56–63.
17. Melnick G, De Leon G. Clarifying the nature of therapeutic community treatment: a survey of essential elements. J Subst Abus Treat. 1999;16:307.
18. Moncrieff JD, Drummond DC, Candy B, et al. Sexual abuse in people with alcohol problems: a study of prevalence of sexual abuse and its relationship to drinking behavior. Br J Psychiatry. 1996;169:355–60.
19. Najavits LM, Weiss RD, et al. The link between substance abuse and posttraumatic stress disorder in women: a research review. Am J Addict. 1997;6:273–83.

20. Najavits L. Seeking safety: a treatment manual for PTSD and substance abuse. New York: The Guilford Press; 2002.
21. Perfas F. Deconstructing the therapeutic community: a handbook for addiction professionals. New York: Hexagram Publishing; 2012.
22. Perfas F. Therapeutic community: past, present, and moving forward. New York: Hexagram Publishing; 2014.
23. Perfas F. Therapeutic community: as a social system. New York: Hexagram Publishing; 2018.
24. Perfas FB, Spross S. Why concept-based therapeutic community can no longer be called drug-free. J Psychoactive Drugs. 2007;39(1):69–79.
25. Raimo S. Democratic and concept-based therapeutic communities and the development of community therapy. In: Rawlings B, Yates R, editors. Therapeutic communities for the treatment of drug users. London: Jessica Kingsley Publishers; 2001. p. 43–56.
26. Stringer C. Lone survivors: how we came to be the only humans on earth. New York: Times Books; 2012.
27. Rice C, Mohr CD, Del Boca FK, Mattson ME, et al. Self-reports of physical, sexual and emotional abuse in alcoholism treatment sample. J Stud Alcohol. 2001;61:114–23.
28. Van der Kolk B. The body keeps the score. New York: Penguin Books; 2014.
29. Wiet S. Origins of addiction predictably embedded in childhood trauma: a neurobiological review. J Korean Acad Child Adolesc Psychiatry. 2017;8(1):4–13.
30. Yablonsky L. Synanon: the tunnel back. New York: Macmillan; 1965.

The Opioid Epidemic

4

Rachel Knight

Introduction

The United States is undeniably in the throes of a drug crisis. There were 70,000 drug overdose deaths in the United States in 2017, an increase of nearly 10% compared to the prior year. Opioids account for 68% of these deaths. Opioids are designed to reduce pain, but are often abused because of their potential to induce euphoria. They also act on receptors that influence respiration and, for this reason, can be lethal in overdose.

Throughout the twenty-first century, the United States has seen escalating rates of opioid misuse, abuse, addiction, as well as fatal overdoses. Opioid-related deaths are six times higher than in 1999, and it is now estimated that opioids overdoses will result in the death of about 130 Americans daily [23]. Despite national efforts to halt this trajectory, we continue to see skyrocketing death tolls, which recently has been driven by the introduction of illicit fentanyl. It is clear we have yet to uncover a meaningful solution, and it is frightening to consider what the future holds. A better understanding of the problem is paramount to developing a viable solution.

R. Knight (✉)
New York Presbyterian – Weill Cornell Medical Center,
New York, NY, USA
e-mail: rnk9002@nyp.org

J. D. Avery, K. A. Kast (eds.), *The Opioid Epidemic and the Therapeutic Community Model*, https://doi.org/10.1007/978-3-030-26273-0_4

In order to better understand the modern opioid epidemic, this chapter will explore the evolution of opioid use in the United States. A close examination of the United States' complex history with treating pain, largely rooted in good intentions, lays the foundation for understanding the interrelated explanations for the modern-day opioid epidemic. More specifically, we will see how the healing profession became heavily reliant on prescription opioids to liberally treat all types of pain. This had unintended consequences; in the last two decades, unprecedented access to prescription opioid medication has contributed to a nationwide epidemic of drug-related misuse, diversion, and mortality and represents the start of the modern-day opioid epidemic. We will lastly consider what has sustained this problem since 2010, when pushes to decrease prescription opioid access began. Attempts to mitigate the problem led to unexpected, devastating consequences, in particular a resurgence of heroin use and the more recent and frightening increase in high-potency alternatives that are often illegal and highly lethal.

The Epidemic Is a Worldwide Problem but the United States Suffers the Most

The opioid epidemic is a global problem, but the scale of the problem is worse in United States. While not the only issue, the most publicized aspect of the opioid epidemic is opioid overdose deaths, and this statistic helps to frame the scope of the epidemic. The United States had over 45,000 opioid-related deaths in 2017, more than any other country and nearly three times the second most affected country globally (Fig. 4.1). Even after controlling for population size, the United States still rates unfavorably, with 15 opioid-related deaths per 100,000 people – again highest in the world and two times higher than the next closest country (Fig. 4.2). Moreover, the United States ranks number two in the world when looking at the share of deaths in the country that come from opioid use (Fig. 4.3).

Since the turn of the century, rates of opioid overdose deaths in United States have climbed at drastic rates compared to other developing nations (Fig. 4.4). There is no single explanation for why the United States is such an outlier; however, a major factor

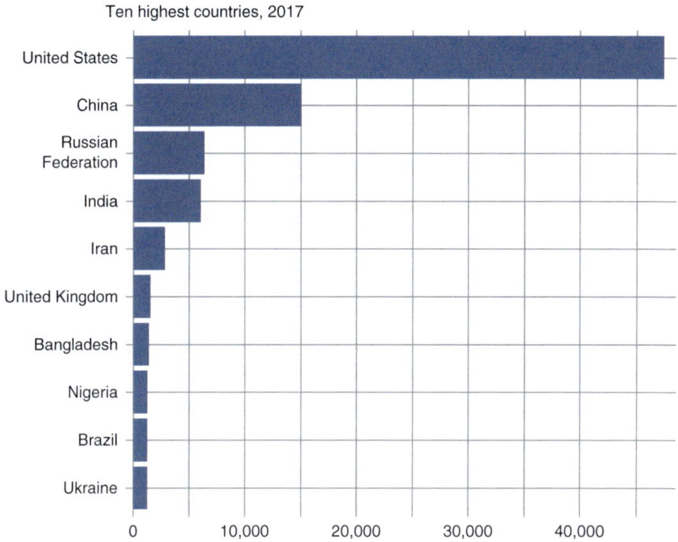

Fig. 4.1 Number of deaths from opioid use (Source: Global Burden of Disease Study 2017)

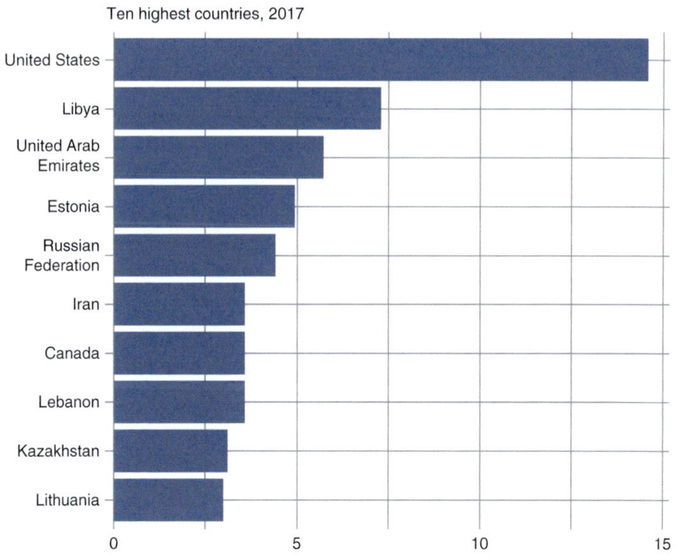

Fig. 4.2 Number of deaths from opioid use per 100,000 people (Source: Global Burden of Disease Study 2017)

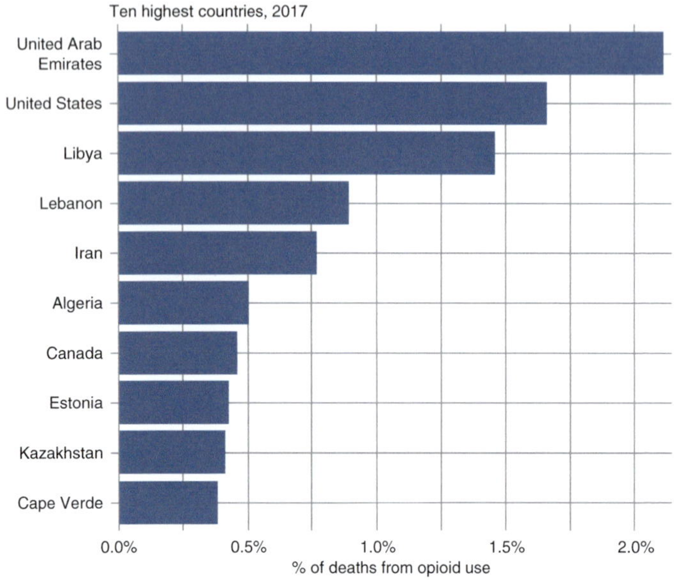

Fig. 4.3 Percentage of deaths from opioid use (Source: Global Burden of Disease Study 2017)

is the inconsistencies in access to prescription opioids around the world. Government policy and local law vary country to country which results in differing levels of access to opioids. Global inequalities in prescription opioid availability are well documented, and an estimated 5.5 billion people currently live in countries with profoundly limited access [17]. In contrast, the United States and Canada both rank in the top two for highest per capita opioid use and together consume the majority of the world's supply of the strongest prescription opioids. This is accompanied by a more disturbing statistic: mortality from prescription opioids seems to be an epidemic relatively unique to North America [11]. It is important to recognize that the opioid epidemic is, in many ways, a by-product of medical care itself. Insufficient pain management is associated with negative health effects, and opioids are undoubtedly effective analgesics and are used with good intentions in mind [20] People aged 12 or older

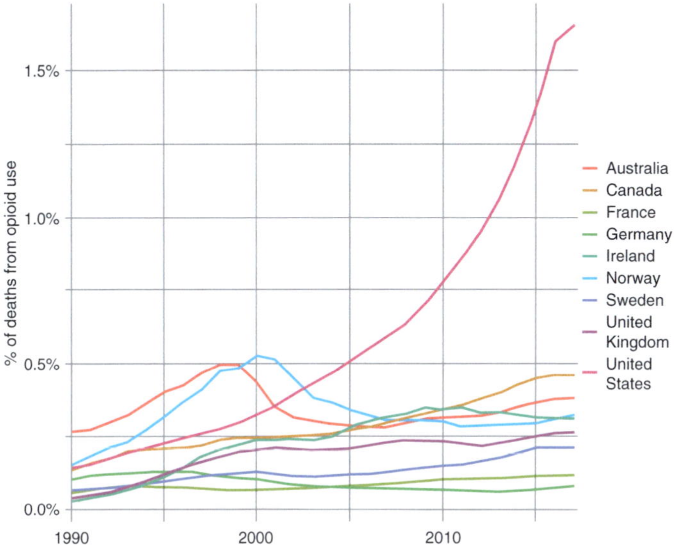

Fig. 4.4 Percentage of deaths from opioid use (Source: Global Burden of Disease Study 2017)

who misused prescription pain relievers in the past year cited relief of physical pain as the most common reason for misuse [18]. It is not surprising then that pain, and the desire to treat it, is the bedrock upon which our current crisis rests.

History of Pain Management Before the 1990s

While pain is a complex phenomenon that until recently has been poorly understood, remedies for pain have long been a part of the canon of medical knowledge. Opiates have been used both medicinally and recreationally for centuries. In 3400 BC, opium was cultivated from the poppy plant, referred to then as the "joy plant." Hippocrates first acknowledged the analgesic and sedative properties for medical use in 460 BC. Once it made its way to Europe, opium was isolated in alcoholic solution to create laudanum – used liberally for a variety of different ailments, including pain, despite a poor understanding of what pain was. Prior before the Scientific Revolution, pain was viewed as an emotion, a "passion of the soul." Understanding the reason for pain was an important philosophical and religious question: perhaps it existed as a form of punishment from the gods or a means to legitimize one's own purpose. The physical and mental aspects of pain were a medical problem too: a physician with a desire to alleviate pain also used it as a marker for vitality or even inflicted it to balance out humors [12]. Throughout the nineteenth century came breakthroughs in scientific research, and pain was gradually redefined as a sensation with its own physiologic apparatus and neural basis. This, coupled with the emergence of utilitarian principles to minimize suffering, led to a shifting desire to aggressively manage pain. Throughout the nineteenth century, opiates and cocaine were the standard of treatment for ailments of any severity with no regulation and sparked the discovery of new compounds that could be marketed for profit [2].

In 1804 German pharmacist Friedrich Wilhelm Adam Sertüner extracted an alkaloid from opium and called it morphine, named after the Greek god of dreams. The creation of morphine stimulated widespread medical interest and enabled physicians to prescribe it in regulated dosages for easing pain. Morphine was incredibly potent and powerful, and inherently valuable for treating severe pain. Its effectiveness resulted in commercial production, and soon, morphine was available over the counter and at local pharmacies. It became known as a cure for many maladies – a mainstay for treating less severe ailments ranging from coughs to anxiety. Hand in hand with its power and potency came a risk for withdrawal and dependence. With morphine and other opioids now cheap, easily accessible, and completely legal, people began to self-medicate and misuse the drug.

In effort to mitigate its addictive potential, the Scottish inventor Dr. Alexander Wood created the hypodermic needle in 1853, claiming that direct injection would isolate the specific area of pain and avoid the addictive potential that comes with swallowing or smoking. Unfortunately, injection of purified morphine likely potentiated the addictive qualities as it allowed for rapid acting delivery, and cases of morphine dependence among the general public began to rise [12]. Injectable morphine was also used as a battlefield anesthetic for soldiers injured in the American Civil War; however, it led to a population of veterans dependent on the drug, leading to the term "soldier's disease." It soon became imperative to find nonaddictive alternatives for managing pain that did not compromise quality and strength. In 1874 Bayer chemist Heinrich Dreser, initially attempting to research nonaddictive alternatives for morphine, synthesized a derivative of morphine called diacetylmorphine and named the drug heroin. Although it was ten times more potent than morphine, it was marked as a "nonaddictive" substitute that could alleviate respiratory ailments associated with the leading causes of death at the time – pneumonia and tuberculosis. At this time there was no regulation on the use of opioids; you could buy it at any drug store. However, it turned out that heroin was indeed highly addictive. To get a greater high, people quickly learned to crush and snort it [9, 10]. Of course, recreational use led to a surge in addiction and dependence and a coincident rise in opioid-related hospitalizations in the United States.

By the early 1900s America was facing a serious problem where unregulated opiates were leading to frightening rates of iatrogenic dependence on morphine and exploding street heroin use. In response, legal efforts arose to curb the problem with an approach that unfortunately criminalized addiction. The Harrison Narcotic Act passed in 1914 which required pharmacists and doctors to pay a tax in order to prescribe. A few years later, production and sale of heroin was banned in the United States entirely. The unintended aftermath was a surge in opioid-related crime as those victims of addiction were now reliant on obtaining their opioids from illegal networks. Mothers, fathers, and working class people victim to addiction were labeled as junkies, and those who came to doctors seeking help for unexplained pain were immediately labeled as malingerer or deluded [9, 10]. Physicians grappled with the dichotomy of wanting to treat pain while fearing the potential of sentencing a patient to drug addiction inflicting the misery and loss of autonomy associated with drug addiction itself. This attitude, referred to as "opiophobia," persisted throughout the latter half of the twentieth century [9, 10]. American physicians reserved opioids for those who were determined to be in severe pain that could be explained by something tangible, such as cancer, and even then, treatment with opioids was reserved for the imminently dying, until the final weeks of life. At this point "opiophobia" had created a culture where addiction was viewed as criminal and immoral, and legitimate pain states were going undertreated [2].

This purposeful underutilization of opioid analgesics persisted until about 1980s when the pendulum shifted in the other direction. There came an era of advocacy for more humane pain treatment [9, 10]. In 1986 the WHO published a Cancer Pain Monograph which highlighted undertreated of postoperative and cancer pain in the United States, leading to tangible improvements in the quality of cancer-related pain treatment with prescription opioids [9, 10]. This approach began to inappropriately extend to non-cancer pain. Several small pieces of literature emerged praising the safety and efficacy of opioids prescribed to patients with chronic non-cancer pain. These pieces would become widely cited in new studies as proof that narcotics are a universally safe treatment for chronic pain. Unfortunately, much of the literature that made up the scientific background for liberalizing the use of opioids for nonmalignant pain were based on small retrospective studies or publications that only considered the treatment of acute pain in hospitalized patients in a regimented setting. While stemming from good intentions to ease suffering, this led to the conflation that the treatment for malignant pain must also be good for pain of a different, much more complex origin: the nonmalignant, chronic pain.

In the late 1990s, the American Pain Society launched the "pain as the fifth vital sign campaign," which required physicians to ask every patient about their level of pain using a numerical treatment algorithm. The campaign (which is no longer recommended by the AMA) pushed doctors to equate pain with any other vital sign like blood pressure or temperature and heart rate or respiratory rate. When reducing it to this, it neglects the idea that pain related to chronic back injury is inherently different in etiology and management when compared to that of end-stage cancer. Nevertheless, physicians were mandated by the Joint Commission on Accreditation of Healthcare Organizations to both adequately assess and control pain of any origin. A patient who rated low satisfaction on the rate of pain treatment on a hospital survey could jeopardize the integrity or reaccreditation of that facility or impact the reimbursements of its employees. The result was a heavy reliance on opioid prescriptions that, at the time, were heavily marketed and being pushed as the most effective treatment for all types of pain [7]. There was, and has always been, a moral obligation to ease suffering for the physician, but now, failure to treat patients in severe pain was viewed as inhumane. The Federation of State Medical Boards and DEA promised less regulation and inspection over the prescription of opioids, and a physician's fear of stigma and scrutinization for potentiating the culture of addiction was replaced with a physician's fear of inadequately treating pain [9, 10].

Creating a Culture of Over-Prescribing

The stage was now set for the modern opioid epidemic. The medical community was relying on a pervasive culture of equating quality healthcare with aggressive pain management, and pain management had now become synonymous with prescription opioids. Inevitably there came a parallel surge in pharmaceutical companies heavily promoting opioid analgesics. From 1997 to 2002, prescriptions for morphine, hydromorphone, fentanyl, and oxycodone increased drastically [19]. During this same time period, extended-release OxyContin became incredibly popular. This drug was aggressively marketed and promoted as a nonaddictive formulation of oxycodone and paralleling the "pain as the fifth vital sign" campaign, its sales almost doubled from its first year on the market [13, 19]. Long-acting OxyContin was supposed to prevent misuse by releasing the drug into the system gradually over time; however, people learned to misuse the drug for more potent and rapid effects by crushing and snorting the pill. It is important to realize that misleading marketing by pharmaceutical companies, as well as inappropriate prescribing practices by physicians themselves, contributed significantly to the prescription opioid epidemic. In 2000 the highest marketed dose of OxyContin was doubled from 80 mg to 160 mg and was approved for opioid-tolerant patients [19]. By 2001 OxyContin was the best-selling narcotic pain reliever in the United States and was the most frequently prescribed opioid for treating moderate to severe pain and the more complex and elusive chronic pain [19].

Failure to Understand Addictive Potential and the Downstream Effects of Nonmedical Use and Pill Diversion

The liberal use of opioids for treating all types of pain is problematic because there is no convincing evidence to suggest that opioids are efficacious in treating chronic pain, nor has there been any epidemiological evidence that medical use of opioids has resulted in reductions in chronic pain [15]. Unlike acute pain, chronic pain has a profoundly different than acute pain and is influenced heavily by a multitude of variables including psychiatric disturbances, unique psychological processing, and psychosocial factors. As such, it is no surprise that the treatment of chronic pain is still poorly understood and an area of ongoing controversy. It is also a common problem: of the many Americans who report some form of pain, the prevalence of chronic pain in older adults is more than 40% [21]. Longer duration of prescribing and higher doses of prescriptions both correlate with increasing overdose and addiction rates [21]. As people use opioids repeatedly, tolerance increases significantly. In addition, repeated exposure leads to a learned association of pain with drug relief, which manifest in an urge or craving to use the drug and ultimately leads to a learned association with receipt of the drug and the positive effects. It is not surprising that up to 30% of patients prescribed opioids for chronic pain misuse them, and of these, roughly 10% develop an opioid use disorder [22]. Unfortunately, none of this was well understood in the early 2000s. Looking back, the desire to eradicate pain coupled with deceptive messages regarding the addictive potential of prescription opioids resulted in patients being exposed to increasing numbers of highly addictive medications. And even after 20 years of unconvincing evidence regarding effectiveness of long-term opioid use, last year enough opioid prescriptions were dispensed to supply roughly 60% of the population with a bottle of pills [6, 16].

Other downstream consequences of this culture of overprescribing were an increase in both pill diversion and nonmedical use of prescription opioids. Diversion of prescription opioids involves transferring prescription opioids obtained from a legal channel to an unlawful channel of distribution (theft, resale), which is an enticing alternative for those whose supply of prescription opioids could not keep up with their developing addiction. Diverted markets also are an opportunity for those who do not have a medical need for narcotics to experiment with them for recreational use. Millions of people report the use of opioid medications that are not prescribed for them or that is taken for the positive euphoric experience it causes [3].

More recent survey statistics estimate that roughly 4000 people begin nonmedical use of prescription opioids a day [18]. Certain studies involving teenagers who have experimented with nonmedical prescription opioid use suggest that they carry many misconceived thoughts about prescription opioids and are unaware of the dangers of this class of medications, one example being the exponential increased risk of overdose when used in combination with alcohol. Those who obtain opioids through a diverted opioid using network are also less likely to be informed about overdose awareness and prevention services. The fact that these medications are widely available and also prescribed legitimately for a medical purpose (often to friends or family members) perpetuates an idea that prescription opioids are less dangerous than illicit opioids like heroin. This creates a vulnerable population of opioid users who are at high risk of the adverse effects related to prescription opioid overdose, including death [5]. This further emphasizes how a culture of overprescribing prescription opioids, despite the best of intentions, did little to change the experience of pain in America, but instead opened the floodgates to the modern-day opioid epidemic.

The Switch to Heroin

In 2010 came several efforts designed to curb the culture of prescription opioid abuse. These included education of healthcare professionals about the appropriate use of opioids, prescription drug monitoring programs that limit a patient's ability to obtain excessive prescriptions, and eradicating lucrative clinics or offices that recklessly dispense narcotics without medical cause ("pill mills") [3, 4]. These pushes also coincided with a rebranding of some of the most widely abused narcotics. In 2010 OxyContin and other prescription opioids were reformulated to an abuse-deterrent formula, leading to the intended positive effects of decreased rates of OxyContin abuse and a relative leveling off of deaths related to prescription opioids by 2013 [4]. In areas with more drastic state and local efforts, the diversion and abuse of and death related to prescription opioids have declined or at least plateaued [3]. This underscores the direct relationship between the ease of availability of prescription opioids and the associated adverse outcomes of misuse and overdose deaths [4]. But the opioid epidemic is still rampant, and unfortunately, the well-intentioned efforts to alter prescription opioid access have had unintended consequences.

As of 2011 there has been a well-documented resurgence in heroin use, with corresponding increases in heroin-related overdoses [4]. Changes to an abuse-deterrent formulation have left those addicted to the drugs in need of alternatives. Heroin is a viable alternative because it is cheap and potent, and the illegal heroin market is often far more accessible than the illegal prescription market [19]. Heroin use is not isolated to inner cities or minority populations but is rising among people of all genders, age groups, and income levels [1]. In fact, some statistical studies have shown that some of the sharpest increases in heroin use are among populations with historically low use rates including those who are privately insured or who have a high income and a disturbing doubling of heroin use among young people in their early twenties [10]. The face of today's heroin user may conjure a different image than it once did as recent users of heroin are often recent prescription opioid abusers. Studies indicate that the current population of heroin users initially misused prescription opioids, a pattern dramatically different from heroin users in the 1960s who were more likely to report that heroin was the first opioid that they had ever used [19]. Making the switch from prescription drugs to heroin may be cheaper, but it comes with its own set of risks. While prescription opioids can be abused via insufflation and inhalation but also orally, heroin is very commonly injected or snorted. The switch from prescription opioids to heroin is often associated with a change in route of administration, increasing the risk of long-term infections such as HIV and hepatitis C or B. Heroin is highly potent and, as such, highly addictive and prone to overdose. The lack of standardization of heroin makes the user unaware of the dose or purity of what they are using, and products that may look exactly the same can have drastically different effects, increasing the risk of overdose [5].

Sustaining the Epidemic: Transition from Legal to Illegal and the Rise in Potent Alternatives

While the start of the opioid epidemic was dominated by overdoses from semisynthetic prescription opioids such as oxycodone or OxyContin, the present-day opioid epidemic is fueled by synthetic opioids. These are compounds chemically manufactured in a lab that mimic naturally occurring opioids. Synthetic opioid-associated overdose deaths increased by nearly 220% between the years 2010 and 2015 (Prescription Behavior Surveillance System [23]). The main driver of the surge in synthetic opioid overdose deaths is fentanyl, which is now the most common drug involved in any drug overdose in the United States [8]. Fentanyl is a synthetic opioid that is incredibly powerful – 50–100 times more potent than morphine – and used medically to treat severe pain including like that related to late stage cancer. Legal fentanyl comes in a variety of forms including lozenges and transdermal patches and can easily be diverted for misuse carrying its own dangerous risk for adverse effects. Fentanyl is also produced illicitly and sold on the black market, often mixed with heroin, cocaine, methamphetamine, or other drugs of abuse to increase potency or euphoric effects [9, 10]. Often times the user lacks the knowledge that they are using a combination product. Illicit fentanyl often comes in the form of a powder, making it incredibly difficult to standardize. Adding to the danger is that the dose of fentanyl required to create a pleasurable effect is incredibly small – similar to a few grains of salt – and even the smallest variations in preparation could lead to a fatal dose. DEA reports indicate that illicit fentanyl is readily available on the opioid black market, and rates of state law enforcement confiscating illegal fentanyl are increasing each month in certain geographic areas like the Eastern and Midwestern United States [16].

Recent data show that as law enforcement drug reports for fentanyl increase in a certain geographic area, so do rates of synthetic opioid overdoses, independent of prescription fentanyl rates. This suggests that illicitly manufactured fentanyl is responsible for the vast majority of recent opioid overdoses in the United States (Prescription Behavior Surveillance System [23]). Eradicating these markets has proven incredibly difficult to control, so efforts to improve detection of fentanyl outbreaks and to educate the public on overdose response actions are becoming important initiatives. Current public health warnings are also promoting awareness about carfentanil, a fentanyl-relative and the most potent commercial opioid in the world according to the DEA. Reports of carfentanil have recently surfaced and are causing its own wave of overdoses across the country. Unlike fentanyl, carfentanil is not approved for use in humans because it is highly lethal at very small doses. First responders to drug confiscations who encounter the drug are at risk of respiratory depression just by inhaling some of the airborne powder. Without proper control of the production and supply of these drugs, the new wave of synthetic opioid use has the potential to far surpass the current trends in mortality related to opioid overdoses [14].

Conclusions

Over the past 20 years, the opioid epidemic has evolved significantly. What once began as a desire to ease pain and human suffering has unfortunately had a devastating impact on the country as a whole. The United States' long history of overreliance on pharmacological approaches to pain management, as well as an underestimation about the addictive potential of opioid analgesics, opened the floodgates to the opioid epidemic. Profits generated by this mindset have impacted decisions made by pharmaceutical companies as well as physicians. Despite guidelines and regulations to mitigate access to prescription opioids, death rates from heroin and illicit synthetic opioids continue to soar. Fentanyl presents a new level of danger to the opioid epidemic: once responsible for just 4% of opioid overdose deaths in 2011, fentanyl is now the leading agent involved in all drug overdoses in the United States [8].

The opioid epidemic has already taken millions of lives. It is responsible for tearing families apart and leaving children parentless. It impacts our friends and our co-workers. But the scope of the epidemic expands far beyond what was covered in this chapter. While opioid overdoses are the most dramatic and highly publicized consequence of opioid misuse, there are many other aspects of the opioid epidemic that are also quite devastating but receive less attention such as increased rates of neonatal abstinence syndrome or increases in long-term viral infections as a result of IV drug use [19]. Society as a whole feels the economic burden – predicted to escalate – with an estimate cost of $78.5 billion a year to cover healthcare, addiction treatment, the loss of productivity, and criminal justice involvement. While incredibly imperative, there is a lot of work that must be done before uncovering a solution. Just like there are many interrelated explanations for the opioid epidemic, addressing the crisis means approaching it from many angles. Recommendations include investing in research to better understand the complicated neurobiology of pain and to explore non-opioid interventions for chronic intractable pain states. It is also important to focus on eradicating the illicit markets that allow potent and lethal synthetic opioids to enter the country. There is also opportunity to save the lives of those who are currently battling an opioid use disorder. And now that modern medicine is beginning to embrace addiction as a disease rather than a moral failure, the hope is that advancements in recovery approaches will play a major role in meaningfully changing the opioid epidemic.

References

1. Cicero TJ, Ellis MS, Surratt HL, et al. The changing face of heroin use in the United States: a retrospective analysis of the past 50 years. JAMA Psychiat. 2014;71(7):821–6.
2. Clarke JL, Skoufalos A, Scranton R. The American opioid epidemic: population health implications and potential solutions, report from the National Stakeholder Panel. Popul Health Manag. 2016;19:S1–S10.
3. Compton W, Jones CM, Baldwin CT. Relationship between nonmedical prescription-opioid use and heroin use. N Engl J Med. 2016;374:154–63.
4. Dart RC, Surratt HL, Cicero TJ. Trends in opioid analgesic abuse and mortality in the United States. N Engl J Med. 2015;372:241–8.
5. Frank D, Mateu-Gelabert P, Guarino H, et al. High risk and little knowledge: overdose experiences and knowledge among young adult nonmedical prescription opioid users. Int J Drug Policy. 2015;26(1):84–91.
6. Florence CS, Zhou C, Luo F, et al. The economic burden of prescription opioid overdose, abuse, and dependence in the United States. Med Care. 2016;54(10):901–6.
7. Guy GP, Zhang K, Bohm MK, et al. Vital signs: changes in opioid prescribing in the United States, 2006–2015. Morb Mortal Wkly Rep. 2017;66(697–704):4.
8. Hedegaard H, Brigham B, Trinidad J et al. Drugs most frequently involved in drug overdose deaths: United States, 2011–2016. Center for Disease Control and Prevention National Vital. Statistics Reports. 2018;67(9):1–13.
9. Jones MR, Viswanath O, Peck J, et al. A brief history of the opioid epidemic and strategies for pain medicine. Pain Ther. 2018a;7:13.
10. Jones CM, Einstein EB, Compton WM. Changes in synthetic opioid involvement in drug overdose deaths in the United States, 2010-2016. JAMA. 2018b;319(17):1819–21.
11. King NB, Fraser V, Boikos C, et al. Determinants of increased opioid-related mortality in the United States and Canada, 1990-2013: a systematic review. Am J Public Health. 2014;104(8):e32–42.
12. Meldrum ML. A capsule history of pain management. JAMA. 2003;290(18):2470–5.
13. Meldrum ML. The ongoing opioid prescription epidemic: historical context. Am J Public Health. 2016;106(8):1365–6.
14. O'Connor S. Fentanyl: China's deadly export to the United States. U.S.-China Economic and Security Review Commission. Staff Research Report, 2017.
15. Rosenblum A, Marsch LA, Joseph H, et al. Opioids and the treatment of chronic pain: controversies, current status, and future directions. Exp Clin Psychopharmacol. 2008;16(5):405–16.
16. Rudd RA, Aleshire N, Zibbell JE, et al. Increases in drug and opioid overdose deaths—United States, 2000-2014. Morbid Mortal Wkly. 2016;64:1378.

17. Seya MJ, Gelders SF, Achara OU, et al. A first comparison between the consumption of and the need for opioid analgesics at country, regional, and global levels. J Pain Palliat Care Pharmacother. 2011;25(1):6–18.
18. Substance Abuse and Mental Health Services Administration. Key substance use and mental health indicators in the United States: results from the 2016 National Survey on drug use and health (HHS Publication No. SMA 17–5044, NSDUH Series H-52). Rockville: Center for Behavioral Health Statistics and Quality, Substance Abuse and Mental Health Services Administration; 2017.
19. Skolnick P. Annual review of pharmacology and toxicology the opioid epidemic: crisis and solutions. Annu Rev Pharmacol Toxicol. 2018;58:143–59.
20. Taylor AL. Addressing the global tragedy of needless pain: rethinking the United Nations single convention on narcotic drugs. J Law Med Ethics. 2007;5(4):556–70.
21. Volkow ND, McLellan AT. Opioid abuse in chronic pain-- misconceptions and mitigation strategies. N Engl J Med. 2016;374:1253–63.
22. Vowles KE, McEntee ML, Julnes PS, et al. Rates of opioid misuse, abuse, and addiction in chronic pain: a systematic review and data synthesis. Pain. 2015;156(4):569–76.
23. Wide-ranging online data for epidemiologic research (WONDER). Atlanta: CDC, National Center for Health Statistics; 2017. Available at http://wonder.cdc.gov.

5 Response to the Opioid Epidemic: Current Treatment Models in the United States

Joseph Bravoco

Introduction

As opioid use disorder is classified as a chronic relapsing disorder [11, 15], its treatment requires a long-term approach. As such, it is important to provide an overview of such treatment strategies while clarifying essential terminology. Detoxification (or medically supervised withdrawal), defined as the management of opioid withdrawal symptoms occurring following discontinuation of the substance, primarily addresses the "physical" component of addiction [5, 15] and is often considered the first step in treatment; it is important to point out, though, that detoxification alone needs to be accompanied by longitudinal treatment to fully address the chronic relapsing course of substance addiction [15]. Through administration and implementation of maintenance therapy, including both long-term opioid replacement and psychosocial/supportive treatments, the full syndrome of addiction is appropriately addressed [15]. While no specific combination of treatment modalities has been consistently demonstrated to be superior to others, there is sufficient evidence to conclude that the utilization

J. Bravoco (✉)
New York-Presbyterian Hospital/Weill Cornell Medical Center, New York, NY, USA
e-mail: Job9207@nyp.org

J. D. Avery, K. A. Kast (eds.), *The Opioid Epidemic and the Therapeutic Community Model*, https://doi.org/10.1007/978-3-030-26273-0_5

of multiple treatment modalities is more effective than adherence to a stand-alone treatment [15]. Furthermore, the "ideal" approach is the one that is tailored to a specific patient at a specific time while being sensitive to the sociocultural and psychological factors inherent to treatment [3] and avoiding stigmatizing language or attitudes [17].

Detoxification

It should be emphasized that detoxification alone is only part of the full range of treatment for opioid use disorder [1, 15]. The primary goal of detoxification should focus on safe management of withdrawal phenomena, during which time the patient habituates to an opioid-free state [5, 15]. Opioid detoxification remains, for the vast majority of individuals with heroin use disorder, a pretreatment procedure prior to residential community treatment, outpatient drug-free treatments, and opioid antagonist maintenance therapy [5]. However, while long-term treatment is typically considered the gold standard of ensuring sobriety, minimizing relapse and recidivism, and promoting a substance-free lifestyle, some patients elect to solely undergo detoxification without long-term treatment, either due to the expectation of maintaining abstinence without additional support or, more commonly, significant ambivalence around the decision to remain abstinent [5]. Additionally, while many individuals with substance use disorders may intend to enroll in therapeutic community and antagonist maintenance treatments, the required detoxification and subsequent withdrawal constitute a significant barrier to meeting selection criteria for such treatments [1, 4, 15].

Currently, most approaches to detoxification remain hampered by factors such as high dropout and relapse rates [5]. These include self-detoxification methods ("cold turkey," use of opioids/benzodiazepines, avoidance, distraction) or traditional detoxification methods utilizing methadone (with adjunctive agents, such as alpha-2 agonists), buprenorphine [1, 4, 15], or clonidine [6]. This is likely due to concerns on the part of opioid-dependent individuals of physical discomfort associated with opioid withdrawal. Some patients may attempt medically assisted detoxification, either in inpatient, residential, or outpatient setting, without successfully completing it to simply lower the financial cost of their habit [5]. Even still, those who complete detoxification have an inherently high relapse rate [15]. Such concerns have given rise to techniques known as "ultrarapid" (anesthesia-assisted detoxification) and antagonist induction procedures, such as naltrexone; despite the potential advantages to these techniques, which have been advertised as a "quick and painless" way to manage opioid withdrawal, such procedures are typically expensive and uncommonly covered by insurance, come with significant medical risks, and lack an evidence base supporting effectiveness [1, 4, 15].

While opioid detoxification constitutes an important step in the treatment of opioid use disorder, we will shift our focus to opioid maintenance treatment, considering both pharmacologic and nonpharmacologic approaches.

Opioid Maintenance Treatment

Use of opioids for maintenance pharmacotherapy traces its roots back to the 1960s, beginning with the advent of methadone administration [1, 14, 15]. Methadone maintenance has demonstrated marked reduction in mortality, decreased illicit substance use, decreased rates of HIV seroconversion, diminished co-occurring criminal activity/prosecution, and overall increased social engagement, improving patients' quality of life. Notwithstanding its demonstrated success, methadone maintenance remains highly stigmatized and remains separate from mainstream medical practice, in large part due to clinicians' poor understanding of its practicality and implementation [1, 14, 15]. With the advent of buprenorphine in 2002, clinicians were afforded the advantage of office-based treatment and possibility of destigmatizing medication-assisted treatment for opioid use disorder. However, due to restrictions on storage and record keeping and special licensing requirements, barriers still persist for many, even within the mental health field.

Methadone Maintenance Treatment

Methadone is a long-acting mu-opioid receptor agonist. It is dispensed within specialized settings, such as methadone maintenance clinics. The induction phase is considered the most important phase of treatment, with most patients requiring 80–120 mg/d of methadone [8]. The starting dose must be significantly lower, with steady state reached gradually over a period of weeks, particularly within the first 10–14 days, with some studies reporting deaths during this time when induction doses are supratherapeutic (>50 mg) and/or the patient is also taking sedatives. In fact, nearly 42% of drug-related deaths during methadone maintenance treatment occur within the first week [8]. Current federal regulations mandate that the initial dose not exceed 30 mg and can be lower in patients with lower-than-expected tolerance. Steady-state levels are typically reached after four to five half-lives (methadone's average half-life ranging from 24 to 36 hours). Given that a significant portion of the previously administered dose remains within lipid stores, as a consequence of methadone's highly lipophilic nature, daily methadone levels increase even in the absence of dose adjustment.

Once a stable dose has been established, the maintenance phase of treatment begins. The great majority of patients are well maintained on daily dose range of 80–120 mg, with a large subset of patients remaining at their original maintenance dose for several years. Factors such as dose level and treatment duration should be individualized and are impacted by a patient's desire to remain on treatment, determination of risk of relapse, and presence/absence of adverse effects. It is important to note that mean, random, or trough levels are not definitive measures for dose adequacy; still, blood level assays are helpful in assessing possible drug-drug interactions and even in cases where a patient may require a split dose due to ultrarapid metabolism [8].

Care must be taken in light of methadone's metabolism by CYP450 system. Certain medications that induce CYP450 may shorten the duration of action and minimize the effect of methadone (such as phenytoin, carbamazepine, rifampicin, phenobarbital, and certain HAART medications), ultimately resulting in a withdrawal phenomenon. Furthermore, drugs that inhibit CYP450 activity (such as ciprofloxacin, fluconazole, erythromycin, cimetidine, and fluvoxamine) will result in longer duration of drug effect and higher potential of methadone side effects and possible overdose. Additionally, clinicians should carefully monitor patients' cardiac rhythm, given the possibility of QT interval prolongation and cardiac arrhythmias (notably, torsade des pointes).

Inherent to methadone maintenance treatment is the potential for diversion, typically in the context of pain management. Recent increases in methadone abuse have paralleled that of prescription opioids [8]. Furthermore, recent data indicates that deaths secondary to methadone overdoses have exceeded deaths from heroin overdoses in certain states since 2002 [8].

Buprenorphine Maintenance Treatment

Buprenorphine is a partial mu-receptor opioid agonist, approved by FDA in 2002, for treatment of opioid dependence. Buprenorphine comes in two sublingual formulations: buprenorphine alone, which is typically used in controlled settings (inpatient medically supervised withdrawal) or in pregnancy, and a combination of buprenorphine and naloxone (Suboxone), with the addition of naloxone to discourage injected diversion and misuse, which is preferred for office-based treatment [8].

Similar to methadone, buprenorphine has both slow onset and long duration of action. It differs in its partial mu-agonism, which affords a maximal dose-effect ceiling without resulting in significant respiratory depression. Moreover, due to its partial agonist property with strong receptor affinity, patients will experience rapid onset of opioid withdrawal. Therefore, it is recommended to provide first dose when the patient is already in opioid withdrawal, between 2 and 4 mg and not exceeding 8 mg [8]. Subsequently, the dose can be rapidly titrated over the next 3 days to minimize withdrawal; average daily dose typically ranges from 16 to 20 mg, prescribed in a single dose. Doses exceeding 32 mg/d have not demonstrated additional maintenance benefit [8]. If the patient requires supervised dosing, buprenorphine can be given every other day or three times a week, while maintaining the total weekly dose [8].

Certain restrictions apply to the office-based setting, as set forth in the Drug Addiction Treatment Act of 2000 [14]. Specifically, these restrictions include census, type of medication, and rules regarding proper storage and record keeping [14]. If buprenorphine is administered in an opioid treatment program, federal regulatory restrictions overseeing dispensing of methadone similarly apply, with one notable exception being the time-in-treatment regulations that apply to take-home methadone doses and no longer apply for buprenorphine.

Recent systematic reviews have demonstrated that buprenorphine is superior to methadone in patient retention [8]. However, neither medication has been shown to be more effective in regard to various other clinical outcomes. Buprenorphine offers an advantage for those patients who prefer to have opioid maintenance treatment prescribed by their physician in a private office without the requirement of receiving medication from a counselor-staffed opioid treatment clinic [12, 13, 14, 17]. Additionally, rates of buprenorphine abuse in the United States remain low, with one study finding 77 reported cases per 1000 prescriptions in 18 regional poison-control centers from 2003 to 2005 [3, 15].

Naltrexone Maintenance Treatment

Naltrexone is a pure opioid antagonist, which was approved for opioid dependence treatment by the FDA in 1984. As a result of having a higher affinity for mu receptors than heroin, morphine, or methadone, naltrexone will displace such drugs from their respective receptors, nullifying their effects; this gives rise to withdrawal symptoms in patients who have not been abstinent from short-acting opioids for 7 days and from long-acting opioids for at least 10 days [15]. Oral naltrexone should be initiated following this acute withdrawal period; initial dose is typically 25 mg on the first day, then 50 mg daily, or an equivalent of 350 mg weekly divided into 3 doses (100, 100, and 150 mg). There is no documented abuse potential and no evidence of withdrawal symptoms from naltrexone upon discontinuation. Naltrexone is particularly effective in highly motivated opioid-dependent patients; however, for those who may be less motivated and for whom medication adherence presents a concern, oral naltrexone is associated with poor retention in treatment [8]. Recent introduction of Naltrexone-XR (Vivitrol), an extended-release monthly injectable approved by the FDA in 2010 to treat opioid dependence, has shown an increase in opioid-free days, enhanced treatment retention, and significant reduction in cravings.

Heroin Maintenance

Heroin maintenance involves providing prescribed heroin as part of a harm-reduction strategy for heroin-dependent patients who have failed other treatment interventions. Initial data was promising, showing that heroin maintenance produced superior outcomes to methadone maintenance based on employment, quality of family and social relationships, medical and psychiatric states, and reduction in nondrug criminal activity [15]. However, prior studies (including a Cochrane systematic review of effectiveness in 2006) resulted in inconclusive findings concerning treatment retention, relapse to street-heroin use, criminal behavior, and overall social functioning, which may have been due to heterogeneity of interventions and outcome measures [15]. For patients who have not been successful with prior trials of methadone or buprenorphine maintenance, heroin maintenance may be indicated.

Other Pharmacologic Approaches

Novel anti-addiction medications, such as new formulations of buprenorphine and naltrexone, off-label uses of clonidine and tramadol, and not-yet-FDA-approved medications such as N-methyl-D-aspartic acid (NMDA) or corticotropin-releasing hormone (CRH) receptor antagonists, furnish a new wave of optimism in the hopes of improving outcomes in opioid maintenance treatment. Use of oral naltrexone at ultralow doses, which have been associated with fewer withdrawal symptoms during methadone-assisted taper, possibly through preventing or counteracting likely receptor changes associated with chronic opioid receptor agonist use, has been proposed [5, 15]. Immunotherapies have mass appeal because of their lack of addiction liability, optimized side effect produced, and possibility of long-term protection against substance use [5, 15]. Initial development of a bivalent vaccine against morphine/heroin has been described in animal models, with vaccinated rats developing antibodies against heroin that antagonized its reinforcing effects [5, 15]. While this certainly has promise, a successful antidrug vaccine would not address the underlying reasons for and consequences of addiction, thereby limiting its usefulness as a stand-alone treatment [15].

Non-pharmacologic Interventions

Psychosocial interventions are part of an integrated approach to treatment of opioid use disorder and play a key role in methadone maintenance treatment [9, 10]. Behavioral therapies, such as CBT and contingency management, can enhance the effectiveness of medication-assisted treatment, though have also been shown to be effective alone [15]. Needle exchange programs have been consistently shown to be both clinically and cost effective in reducing rates of HIV transmission, without any convincing evidence for unintended negative consequences, such as increases in illicit drug use initiation, duration, or injection frequency. Additionally, evidence suggests that needle exchange programs likely incentivize entry into drug-treatment programs and contact with primary care providers [5, 15].

Addiction treatment in the United States occurs across a spectrum of levels of care. The American Society of Addiction Medicine's (ASAM) patient placement criteria attempt to match patients to five levels: (1) early intervention, (2) outpatient treatment, (3) intensive outpatient or partial hospitalization treatment, (4) residential or inpatient treatment, and (5) medically managed intensive inpatient treatment. Six dimensions are assessed for individual patients in determining the appropriate level of care: (a) acute intoxication/withdrawal state, (b) medical comorbidity, (c) psychiatric comorbidity, (d) readiness for change, (e) potential for relapse, and (f) current recovery/living environment [4]. Regarding the level of care appropriate for an individual patient with opioid use disorder, the degree of impairment across these six dimensions—whether due to the severity of substance use, comorbid psychiatric disorders, socioeconomic instability, homelessness, and involvement in the legal system, among other complicating factors—correlates with the required intensity of treatment. Extrapolating results of studies for alcohol and mixed substance use disorders, inpatient or residential treatment settings show greater benefit for the more impaired patients [4].

Length of stay (LOS) also affects outcomes, with longer LOS correlating with lower substance-use-related symptoms, better psychosocial functioning, and lower readmission rates; however, these benefits of long LOS appear to occur only for the more impaired population [2, 4]. Data from recent outcome studies, for longer LOS for patients requiring residential treatment, appear to correlate with notably better outcomes in rates of substance reuse, reintegration into workforce and vocational pursuits, engagement in illicit activity, and improvement in comorbid psychiatric disorders [8].

Despite the evidence for longer LOS in more impaired patients, payer reimbursement for inpatient/residential treatment settings has incentivized shorter LOS over time, given the relative cost effectiveness without loss of treatment benefit for less impaired patients [4]. This has led to 30- or 60-day LOS being "typical" for most treatment centers, and the term "short-term rehab" is appropriately applied. The 90-day (or more) LOS known to be more effective for more impaired patients has become far less common in our current system of care (outside the correctional system) due to this change in reimbursement, leading to a crisis for patients who would benefit from more time in treatment.

Access to treatment and appropriate linkage of care remain cornerstone issues in providing high-quality opioid maintenance treatment to patients in need [7]. Methadone maintenance treatment, for example, reaches only 15–20% of those requiring treatment [7, 8]. Recent legislations, including the Drug Addiction Treatment Action (DATA) of 2000 and Health Parity and Addiction Equity Act in 2008, have focused efforts on legalizing office-based opioid maintenance treatments to private practice physicians and improving access to treatment for mental illness and addiction, respectively.

The high prevalence of medical and psychiatric comorbidities in patients with opioid use disorder is well-known within both the medical and lay communities. Still, current treatment for those with comorbid conditions remains poorly coordinated, given continued reliance on a parallel approach model. Further attention should be paid to instituting a collaborative, multidisciplinary system that allows mental health clinicians, primary care providers, and addiction specialists to work in a more integrated fashion and practice optimized patient-centered clinical care. Linkage of substance abuse and primary care providers has a number of benefits, including widening access to both forms of care, reducing stigma of substance use disorder among medical providers, and paving the way for greater parity of reimbursements for substance abuse services [16]. Moreover, this approach would appear to seemingly increase health-care system efficiency and decrease health-care costs by minimizing the need for emergency room and hospital visits among methadone maintenance and long-term residential patients, instead of streamlining this care through primary care and/or off-site referrals [3].

Conclusion

Current treatment models for opioid use disorder include detoxification and maintenance therapies, as well as non-pharmacologic methods. Methadone and buprenorphine remain the mainstay of treatments, with slight differences in the delivery and long-term provision of each that may inform suitability for certain patients [8]. Novel anti-addiction medications and long-acting formulations of buprenorphine appear to represent the next wave of pharmacologic approaches to opioid maintenance treatment. Psychosocial interventions, both when combined with pharmacologic methods and by themselves, play a significant role in improving treatment outcomes and should be considered an integral part of any treatment approach for opioid use disorder [15]. Needle exchange programs have significant value in harm-reduction properties and have proven cost effectiveness [5, 15]. Continued legislative and institutional efforts to enhance access to treatment and linkage to care are necessary to destigmatize substance use and provide optimal, well-integrated treatment across medical and psychiatric specialties.

References

1. Avery J, Barnhill J. Co-occurring mental illness and substance use disorders: a guide to diagnosis and treatment. Arlington: American Psychiatric Publishing; 2017.
2. Center for Behavioral Health Statistics and Quality. Key substance use and mental health indicators in the United States: results from the 2015 national survey on drug use and health. NoSMA 16-4984, NSDUH Ser H-51. 2016;7(1):877–726.
3. Friedman PD, McCullough D, Saitz R. Screening and intervention for illicit drug abuse: a national survey of primary care physicians and psychiatrists. Arch Intern Med. 2001;161:248–51.
4. Finney JW, Moos RH, Wilbourne PL. Effects of treatment setting, duration, and amount on patient outcomes. In: Ries RK, Miller SC, Saitz R, Fiellin DA, editors. American Society of Addiction Medicine The ASAM principles of addiction medicine. 5th ed. Philadelphia: Wolters Kluwer Health and Lippincott Williams & Wilkins; 2014.
5. Galanter M, Kleber HD. The American psychiatric publishing textbook of substance abuse treatment. 4th ed. Washington D.C: American Psychiatric Publishing; 2008.
6. Geller G, Levine DM, Mamon JA, et al. Knowledge, attitudes, and reported practices of medical students and house staff regarding the diagnosis and treatment of alcoholism. JAMA. 1989;262(21):3115–20.
7. Gryczynski J, Schwartz RP, O'Grady KE, et al. Understanding patterns of high-cost health care use across different substance user groups. Health Aff (Millwood). 2016;35(1):12–9.
8. Herron AJ, Brennan TK. The ASAM essentials of addiction medicine. 2nd ed. Philadelphia: Wolters Kluwer; 2015.
9. Humphreys K. Avoiding globalisation of the prescription opioid epidemic. Lancet. 2017;390:437–9.
10. Ianucci R, Sanders K, Greenfield S. A 4-year curriculum on substance use disorders for psychiatry residents. Acad Psychiatry. 2009;33(1):60–6.

11. Koob GF, Vokow ND. Neurocircuitry of addiction. Neuropsychopharmacology. 2010;35:217–38.
12. Miller NS, Sheppard LM, Colenda CC, et al. Why physicians are unprepared to treat patients who have alcohol- and drug-related disorders. Acad Med. 2001;76:410–8.
13. Polydorou S, Gunderson EW, Levin FR. Training physicians to treat substance use disorders. Curr Psychiatry Rep. 2008;10(5):399–404.
14. Renner JA, Levounis P, LaRose AT. Office-based Buprenorphine treatment of opioid use disorder. 2nd ed. Arlington: American Psychiatric Association Publishing; 2018.
15. Ruiz P, Strain S. Substance abuse: a comprehensive textbook. 5th ed. Philadelphia: Wolters-Kluwer; 2011.
16. Samet JH, Friedmann P, Saitz R. Benefits of linking primary medical care and substance abuse services: patient, provider, and society perspectives. Arch Intern Med. 2001;161(1):85–91.
17. Van Boekel LC, Brouwers EPM, Van Weeghel J, et al. Stigma among health professionals towards patients with substance use disorders and its consequences for healthcare delivery: systematic review. Drug Alcohol Depend. 2013;131(1–3):23–35.

6 Target Population: Treatment-Resistant Opioid Use Disorder and the Role of Therapeutic Communities

Kristopher A. Kast

Introduction

This chapter will focus on the population of patients with opioid use disorder (OUD) who may benefit from increasing access to the therapeutic community (TC) model in the larger system of care in the United States. Of all patients with OUD, only a minority receive appropriate medication-assisted treatment (MAT) with methadone, buprenorphine, or extended-release naltrexone. [12, 17] Efforts to increase access to these effective interventions are appropriate and much needed. However, MAT and harm-reduction interventions do not lead to remission or risk reduction for all OUD patients [36]. A significant group continues opioid use with its grave risks despite our first-line treatments. *Yes*, we need to expand access to MAT and harm-reduction interventions, *and* we need to diversify the available treatment modalities for more severely impaired patients and those not currently engaged. Further, MAT and TCs are not exclusive of each other—though there are historical roots to their apparent segregation [2].

K. A. Kast (✉)
Payne Whitney Clinic of New York-Presbyterian,
Weill Cornell Medical College, New York, NY, USA
e-mail: kak9100@nyp.org

J. D. Avery, K. A. Kast (eds.), *The Opioid Epidemic and the Therapeutic Community Model*, https://doi.org/10.1007/978-3-030-26273-0_6

Increased attention to additional treatment approaches for OUD is needed amidst the current opioid crisis. The TC model has been shown to be effective and offers a unique treatment frame for patients considered "treatment resistant," yet it is rarely considered an option in the United States and has not been included in the federal response to the opioid crisis.

"Treatment-Resistant" Opioid Use Disorder and the Treatment Gap

"Treatment resistant" is a common term in the psychiatric treatment of affective and psychotic disorders. It broadly refers to a quality of the neurobiological syndrome, specifically its poor response to first-line treatments. The historical and culturally entrenched stigmatization and moralization of the addiction syndrome may lead to a misinterpretation of "treatment resistant" if it is applied to patients with substance use disorders—"treatment-resistant opioid use disorder" may easily be misread as a patient's volitional (or unconsciously motivated) "resistance" to treatment, or a free choice to avoid treatment and continue problematic substance use. This is not what is meant in this chapter.

Treatment-resistant OUD should refer to a poor response to standard-of-care treatments (specifically MAT), emphasizing a quality of an individual's neurobiological syndrome. Identifying a patient's OUD as treatment resistant should include an assessment of individualized and clinically relevant outcomes, including symptom reduction, engagement in treatment and treatment dropout, amount and frequency of opioid use, related health outcomes (such as infectious disease transmission and obstetrical complications), emergency medical service utilization, criminality and legal-system involvement, housing status, quality of and engagement with a social support network, and employment. An individual patient's treatment response or resistance will include a unique profile across these domains with different significance attributed to each outcome according to shared treatment goals between the patient and treatment team.

Outcome data from clinical trials for MAT show how common suboptimal response to standard-of-care treatments is in the OUD population. Approximately 50–65% of patients randomized to buprenorphine or extended-release naltrexone in the X:BOT study experienced relapse over 24 weeks of follow-up [18]. For extended-release naltrexone, the induction barrier (treatment dropout due to intolerable initiation of the mu-opioid antagonist) led to 28% of patients discontinuing medication (89% of whom relapsed); this is especially meaningful for patients who are unable to receive or object to agonist therapy, showing greater vulnerability to early treatment dropout, relapse, and its sequelae. In this study, treatment retention was lower than relapse rates, with ~45% of patients remaining engaged in both MAT treatment arms at the end of the trial (modestly lower than other MAT studies, where retention is reported nearer 55–66%; [16, 20, 31, 32, 36]). Aggregating these data, approximately 40–55% of patients studied in our best MAT clinical trials do not remain in treatment by study completion—the OUD syndrome in this group may be considered resistant to our current gold-standard treatments.

Treatment resistance in addiction is also distinct from the "treatment gap." In 2017, only 19.3% of individuals with substance use disorder in the United States received any addiction treatment (and only 12.2% received treatment in a specialty facility) highlighting a significant group, >80% of individuals with an addiction syndrome, who received no treatment. This unengaged group is the appropriate target of interventions meant to increase access to gold-standard MAT and increase motivation for change. In this group, only 5.5% perceive a need for treatment and of those who do believe they need treatment, and 40% are not ready to stop using, highlighting an important attitudinal barrier to accessing care that may be amenable to motivational interviewing or related interventions. Additionally, 33% had no health insurance and were unable to pay for treatment.

Our current approach to the treatment-resistant population and those in the treatment gap is harm reduction focused. These include increasing availability and training in the use of naloxone rescue kits to reverse opioid overdose, needle-exchange programs, and supervised injection sites [34]. These are effective from a public health perspective, reducing mortality from opioid overdose and infectious disease transmission rates. However, additional treatment modalities targeting the full range of opioid use disorder outcomes are needed for this group.

The therapeutic community is a well-established and evidence-based treatment modality with unique mechanisms of action that may either augment current gold-standard MAT or serve as monotherapy for patients with demonstrated treatment resistance (or those who object to medication, or for whom our available medications are contraindicated). Additionally, in some models (including the *San Patrignano* community), treatment is provided at no cost to the patient, further reducing perceived barriers to care.

Unique Characteristics of Therapeutic Community Populations

The population served by modern TCs typically present with characteristics that have been identified as poor prognostic indicators for addiction treatment, and often these patients have multiple exclusion criteria for most clinical trials of MAT. Individuals with OUD in TCs commonly have multiple comorbid substance use disorders, most frequently cocaine, cannabis, alcohol, and tobacco. Psychiatric comorbidity is frequent, usually anxiety spectrum and personality disorders, including antisocial, borderline, histrionic, schizotypal, and avoidant traits. Most have a poor work history, with two-thirds not employed full time over the year preceding treatment, and significant criminality with a majority having prior arrests and legal action [6, 7].

Individuals thought to be particularly well suited for referral to TCs have evidence of a life in crisis, including felt anxiety around the risk of serious harm or death due to continued opioid use and/or identified losses due to substance use—thus, a group with some conscious motivation for treatment who are likely to be help seeking in clinical settings. They have demonstrated an impaired ability to maintain treatment goals (reduced use, abstinence, criminal recidivism, etc.) despite prior treatment episodes—that is, there is evidence of treatment resistance. Grave social or interpersonal dysfunction with few relationships and little-to-no employment are also common [13, 14]. Housing status may also be particularly important to consider in thinking about those patients who would benefit from the TC model, with homelessness or tenuous housing indicating potential benefit [23].

These characteristics of TC populations highlight their unique niche within the system of care for patients with addiction. TCs serve individuals who are poorly represented in our MAT clinical trials (due to significant comorbidity and adverse life circumstances) and evidence treatment resistance.

Effectiveness of Therapeutic Communities for the Treatment-Resistant Opioid Use Disorder Population

Significant evidence from large-scale naturalistic field effectiveness studies, single-program controlled studies, randomized-controlled trials, meta-analyses, and cost-benefit analyses support TCs as effective, cost-saving interventions for more impaired patients [8, 28, 33]. Patient outcomes measured include sustained abstinence, reduced drug use, criminal behavior, and employment; cost-benefit analyses include healthcare-related costs and carbon footprint of treatment [21]. The major moderator of response to TC-based intervention is retention in treatment and longer length of stay [3, 7, 8, 28]. Notably, some authors have called into question the quality of evidence supporting TCs' efficacy, often excluding significant field effectiveness studies in exclusive favor of randomized-controlled trials [4, 19, 29]. However, the utility of effectiveness (as opposed to efficacy) studies in treatment-resistant clinical populations and interventions whose complexity rivals that of a university education should not be discounted—especially given the dearth of evidence for treatments targeting a patient population that is largely excluded from MAT clinical trials or difficult to study outside of naturalistic field effectiveness designs [6].

Unique Mechanisms of Therapeutic Efficacy

The active therapeutic component of the TC model is an empirical question under investigation. There is evidence for the following mediators of change:

1. Increasing capacity for responsible agency
2. Imparting a sense of social belongingness
3. Productive pattern of corrective "pull-ups" given and received in social learning
4. Increasing identification with recovery over substance use
5. Cognitive schema change toward TC-based "right living"
6. Increasing mentalization capacity and reflective functioning
7. Educational/occupational habilitation [5, 10, 11, 22, 26, 35]

The TC model shares characteristics of Winnicott's theory of a psychodynamic holding environment (and Bion's theory of psychodynamic containment), fostering a sense of safety and trust necessary for self-exploration and providing optimal frustration of patients' habitual methods of obtaining satisfaction and relieving internal tension [5, 37]. This is thought to allow for a growing capacity to mentalize one's own and others' cognitive-emotional states (moving away from relative alexithymia) and develop reflective functioning necessary for behavior change.

These hypothesized therapeutic mediators may work on different neurobiological substrates than MAT and other evidence-based interventions, including cognitive-behavioral, motivational-interviewing, and relapse-prevention strategies. Analogous synergistic effects of psychotropic medication and psychosocial interventions via divergent underlying neural substrates in the treatment of major depressive disorder suggest the possibility of enhanced efficacy for OUD when combining MAT and TCs, though this remains to be demonstrated and may vary by individual patient characteristics [9].

Further, our increasing neurobiological understanding of the addiction syndrome indicates significant genetic and epigenetic heterogeneity across the population of patients identified as having a substance use disorder [27]. Thus, individuals with OUD likely have diverse underlying neurobiological vulnerabilities that impact response to different treatment modalities, perhaps contributing to treatment resistance. Increasing the complexity of treatment delivered (by combining modalities) has some evidence for efficacy in overcoming less-robust neurobiological response to medication; for example, poor response to naltrexone in alcohol use disorder patients without the A118G polymorphism in the mu-opioid receptor gene, OPRM1, may be overcome by increasing exposure to other psychosocial treatment modalities, though this remains controversial [1, 25]. In the absence of clinically useful markers for response to specific treatment modalities, our system of care will benefit from having a diverse range of treatment modalities targeting multiple underlying neurobiological targets, thus increasing the likelihood that the greatest number of patients will benefit.

Therapeutic Communities and the Treatment Gap

Despite the evidence for effective treatment of a marginalized and treatment-resistant population and the potential for synergistic effects with other evidence-based treatments, TCs have not yet been included in the federal response to the opioid crisis [12]. In contrast, American prisons and correctional settings have shown increasing interest in TC models, with programs in California, Colorado, and Delaware demonstrating less recidivism, increased employment, and better SUD-related outcomes [24]. Although encouraging, this highlights a problematic historical trend in the United States: an overreliance on an under-equipped legal and correctional system to manage mental illness and substance use disorders [15]. Further, these prison-based TCs highlight the importance of ongoing treatment after release, with marked deleterious effects on relevant outcomes when treatment is abruptly discontinued. Thus, availability of non-corrections-based programs is important for these individuals, as well as those not (yet) with legal repercussions to their substance use.

Access to multiple effective treatment modalities with flexible levels of care would seem to increase the likelihood of engaging a diverse population of individuals with opioid and other substance use disorders. This is an important hypothesis, relevant to the >80% of individuals with SUD in the treatment gap [30].

Conclusion

Patients with treatment-resistant opioid use disorder require greater access to other effective treatments, like therapeutic communities, that may complement MAT or serve as monotherapy for those unable to take medication (either due to personal objection or due to medical contraindications). Access to TCs will also diversify available modalities for a largely unengaged population, potentially reducing the treatment gap.

References

1. Anton RF, Oroszi G, O'Malley S, et al. An evaluation of mu-opioid receptor (OPRM1) as a predictor of naltrexone response in the treatment of alcohol dependence: results from the Combined Pharmacotherapies and Behavioral Interventions for Alcohol Dependence (COMBINE) study. Arch Gen Psychiatry. 2008;65(2):135–44.
2. Clark CD. The Recovery Revolution: the battle over addiction treatment in the United States. New York: Columbia University Press; 2017.
3. Condelli WS, Hubbard RL. Relationship between time spent in treatment and client outcomes from therapeutic communities. J Subst Abus Treat. 1994;11:25–33.
4. Cutcliffe JR, Travale R, Richmond MM, Green T. Considering the contemporary issues and unresolved challenges facing Therapeutic Communities for clients with alcohol and substance abuse. Issues Ment Health Nurs. 2016;37(9):642–50.
5. Debaere V, Vanheule S, Inslegers R. Beyond the "black box" of the Therapeutic Community for substance abusers: a participant observation study on the treatment process. Addict Res Theory. 2014;22(3):251–62.
6. DeLeon G. Therapeutic Communities. In: Galanter M, Kleber HD, Brady KT, editors. The American psychiatric publishing textbook of substance abuse treatment. 5th ed; 2015a.

7. DeLeon G. "The Gold Standard" and related considerations for a maturing science of substance abuse treatment. Therapeutic Communities; a case in point. Subst Use Misuse. 2015b;50(8–9):1106–9.
8. DeLeon G. Is the Therapeutic Community an evidenced based treatment? What the evidence says. Int J Therap Commun. 2010;31(2):104–28.
9. DeRubeis RJ, Siegle GJ, Hollon SD. Cognitive therapy vs. medications for depression: treatment outcomes and neural mechanisms. Nat Rev Neurosci. 2008;9(10):788–96.
10. Dingle GA, Stark C, Cruwys T, Best D. Breaking good: breaking ties with social groups may be good for recovery from substance misuse. Br J Soc Psychol. 2015;54(2):236–54.
11. Doogan NJ, Warren K. Semantic networks, schema change, and reincarceration outcomes of therapeutic community graduates. J Subst Abus Treat. 2016;70:7–13.
12. Doherty N, Gottlieb S, McCance-Katz E, Schuchat A, Volkow N. Federal efforts to combat the opioid crisis: a status update on CARA and other initiatives. Testimony to Congressional Senate Committee on Health, Education, Labor & Pensions. Oct 25, 2017. Accessed 1 July 2018 via: https://www.drugabuse.gov/about-nida/legislative-activities/testimony-to-congress/2017/federal-efforts-to-combat-opioid-crisis-status-update-cara-other-initiatives.
13. Finney JW, Moos RH, Wilbourne PL. Effects of treatment setting, duration, and amount on patient outcomes. In: Ries RK, Miller SC, Saitz R, Fiellin DA, editors. American Society of Addiction Medicine The ASAM principles of addiction medicine. 5th ed. Philadelphia: Wolters Kluwer Health and Lippincott Williams & Wilkins; 2014.
14. Kurth DJ. Therapeutic communities. In: Ries RK, Miller SC, Saitz R, Fiellin DA, editors. American Society of Addiction Medicine The ASAM principles of addiction medicine. 5th ed. Philadelphia: Wolters Kluwer Health and Lippincott Williams & Wilkins; 2014.
15. Krawczyk N, Picher CE, Feder KA, Saloner B. Only one in twenty justice-referred adults in specialty treatment for opioid use receive methadone or buprenorphine. Health Aff (Millwood). 2017;36(12):2046–53.
16. Krupitsky E, Nunes EV, Ling W, et al. Injectable extended-release naltrexone for opioid dependence: a double-blind, placebo-controlled, multi center randomized trial. Lancet. 2011;377:1506–13.
17. Larochelle MR, Bernson D, Land T et al. Medication for opioid use disorder after nonfatal opioid overdose and association with mortality. A cohort study. Ann Intern Med. E-publication. 2018.
18. Lee JD, Nunes EV, Novo P, et al. Comparative effectiveness of extended release naltrexone versus buprenorphine-naloxone for opioid relapse prevention (X:BOT): a multicentre, open-label, randomised controlled trial. Lancet. 2018;391(10118):309–18.
19. Malivert M, Fatséas M, Denis C, et al. Effectiveness of therapeutic communities: a systematic review. Eur Addict Res. 2012;18(1):1–11.

20. Manhapra A, Petrakis I, Rosenheck R. Three-year retention in buprenorphine treatment for opioid use disorder nationally in the Veterans Health Administration. Am J Addict. 2017;26(6):572–80.
21. Maughan D, Lillywhite R, Pearce S, Pillinger T, Weich S. Evaluating sustainability: a retrospective cohort analysis of the Oxfordshire therapeutic community. BMC Psychiatry. 2016;16(1):285.
22. Melnick G, De Leon G, Hiller ML, Knight K. Therapeutic communities: diversity in treatment elements. Subst Use Misuse. 2000;35(12–14):1819–47.
23. Milby JB, Schumacher JE, Wallace D, et al. To house or not to house: the effects of providing housing to homeless substance abusers in treatment. Am J Public Health. 2005;95:1259–65.
24. National Institute on Drug Abuse. Research reports: Therapeutic Communities. National Institutes of Health. July 2015.
25. Oslin DW, Leong SH, Lynch KG, et al. Naltrexone vs Placebo for the treatment of alcohol dependence: a randomized clinical trial. JAMA Psychiat. 2015;72(5):430–7.
26. Pearce S, Pickard H. How therapeutic communities work: specific factors related to positive outcome. Int J Soc Psychiatry. 2013;59(7):636–45.
27. Prom-Wormleya EC, Ebejerb J, Dickc DM, Bowers MS. The genetic epidemiology of substance use disor- der: a review. Drug Alcohol Depend. 2017;180:241–59.
28. Sacks S. Overview of therapeutic community outcome research. In: Ries RK, Miller SC, Saitz R, Fiellin DA, editors. American Society of Addiction Medicine The ASAM principles of addiction medicine. 5th ed. Philadelphia: Wolters Kluwer Health and Lippincott Williams & Wilkins; 2014.
29. Smith LA, Gates S, Foxcroft D. Therapeutic communities for substance related disorder. Cochrane Database Syst Rev. 2006;(1):CD005338.
30. Substance Abuse and Mental Health Services Administration (SAMHSA). Key substance use and mental health indicators in the United States: results from the 2017 National Survey on Drug Use and Health (HHS Publication No. SMA 18-5068, NSDUH Series H-53). Rockville, MD: Center for Behavioral Health Statistics and Quality, Substance Abuse and Mental Health Services Administration. 2018. Retrieved from https://www.samhsa.gov/data/.
31. Sullivan MA, Bisaga A, Pavlicova M, et al. A randomized trial comparing extended-release injectable suspension and oral naltrexone, both combined with behavioral therapy, for the treatment of opioid use disorder. Am J Psychiatry. 2019;176(2):129–37.
32. Tanum L, Solli KK, Latif ZE, et al. Effectiveness of injectable extended-release Naltrexone vs Daily Buprenorphine-Naloxone for opioid dependence: a randomized clinical noninferiority trial. JAMA Psychiat. 2017;74(12):1197–205.

33. Vanderplasschen W, Colpaert K, Autrique M, Rapp RC, Pearce S, Broekaert E, Vandevelde S. Therapeutic communities for addictions: a review of their effectiveness from a recovery-oriented perspective. Sci World J. 2013;2013:427817.
34. Volkow ND. Medications for opioid use disorder: bridging the gap in care. Lancet. 2018;391(10118):285–7.
35. Warren K, Hiance D, Doogan N, De Leon G, Phillips G. Verbal feedback in therapeutic communities: pull-ups and reciprocated pull-ups as predictors of graduation. J Subst Abus Treat. 2013;44(4):361–8.
36. Williams AR, Nunes EV, Bisaga A, Pincus HA, Johnson KA, Campbell AN, Remien RH, Crystal S, Friedmann PD, Levin FR, Olfson M. Developing an opioid use disorder treatment cascade: a review of quality measures. J Subst Abus Treat. 2018;91:57–68.
37. Winnicott DW. Playing and reality. 1st ed. New York: Routledge. 2005; 1971.

7 Current Therapeutic Communities Around the World

Phaedon Kaloterakis

Introduction

Therapeutic communities (TCs) by definition are recovery oriented. They focus on the whole person and encourage overall lifestyle change, not simply abstinence from the use of substances. Although they started only 70 years ago, the TC approach has been adopted and applied in more than 65 countries around the world [4].

This broad uptake across diverse sociocultural contexts reflects an intrinsic quality of openness in the TC model. Harold Bridger, one of the pioneers of the Northfield Psychiatric Hospital in England [3, 11], talked in an interview about this openness:

> The basic element in all this work was really not just the activities which people were carrying out, but what people were missing was the idea that it had to contribute to the socialization of people, that people recognized the relationship with others. My idea was to ensure that whilst they could be creative, apart from bearing their creativity, that they could also build this socialization with relation to other people, working with other people. The whole idea… was simply to bring people together. This is more than just being active, doing good things and being a nice family. You had to have what I call the open system

P. Kaloterakis (✉)
KETHEA, European Federation of Therapeutic Communities (EFTC), World Federation of Therapeutic Communities (WFTC), Thessaloniki, Greece
e-mail: phaedon.kal@ketheathess.gr

J. D. Avery, K. A. Kast (eds.), *The Opioid Epidemic and the Therapeutic Community Model*, https://doi.org/10.1007/978-3-030-26273-0_7

> type of community… The idea of a community, of a good community, was not what I was concerned with. It is how do you develop it as an open system with the outside world being as much part of the thing as the inside world. Organizations have to work on open, not closed. Of course you cannot stop being open [15].

In this chapter, I intend to present some highlights of the TC movement as it is spreading around the world and at the same time discuss some of the challenges that TCs will face in the future.

The TC Movement Goes Global

Most people consider Synanon as the first therapeutic community. It is true that Synanon was the pioneer program in dealing with substance use disorders. It was established by Chuck Dederich in Santa Monica, California, in 1958. The endeavor received great coverage from the very start. In 1961, *LIFE* magazine did a lengthy article on Synanon, and a 1965 movie, SYNANON, starring Chuck Connors, glorified the organization [19].

The therapeutic community, as a method though, existed before Synanon. As we already mentioned, there were TCs operating in England right after the end of War World II. Maxwell Jones founded the Industrial Neurosis Unit at the Belmont Hospital, and together with Bion, Bridger, Rickman, and others at Northfield Hospital, Jones was running TCs for traumatized soldiers and the mentally ill [10]. The term therapeutic community was used for the first time in 1946 by Thomas Main, a psychiatrist, in a paper where he presented how staff and clients interact and are mutually involved in a community setting in order to achieve reintegration to society [13].

Even before 1946 though, and during the end of the nineteenth century, there were systematic attempts to operate programs with similar structure to the therapeutic community in order to deal with juvenile delinquency [8]. Mostly educators who disliked the militaristic approach of Baden Powell and the Boy Scouts developed organizations such as the Little Commonwealth and the Boy's Republic [6]. These efforts have many similarities with the TCs of Jones and Dederich (Fig. 7.1).

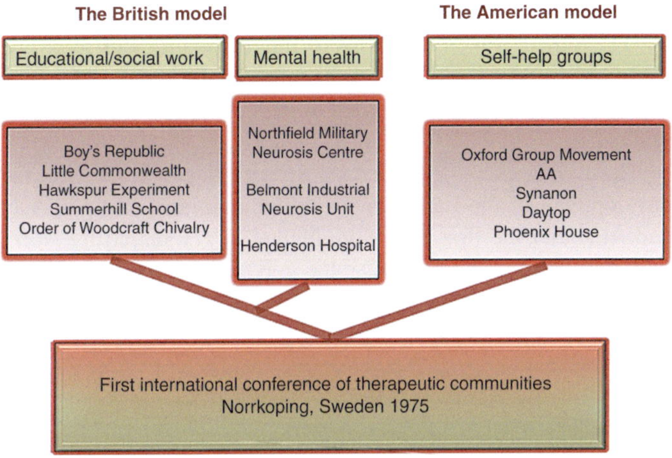

Fig. 7.1 The origins of the therapeutic community

Because these programs were operating within the realms of mental health/self-help and social work/education, they took off quickly. In 1979, George De Leon and Mitchell Rosenthal stated that there were over 300 residential programs in the United States using some variant of the TC model to serve drug abusers, criminal offenders, and others with social disorders [7].

Europe came next. In 1970, Ian Christie established Alpha House in Portsmouth and Griffin Edwards started Phoenix House in London, a few months later. In 1972, Emiliehoeve, the first TC in the Netherlands, was founded by Martien Kooyman [12]. Emiliehoeve assisted in the development of other TCs (Breegweestee, Crowley House, Parkweg House). In Sweden, Lars Breberck founded Vallmotorp, while in Germany, Osterhues, after his visit in New York, founded Daytop, Germany. Erik Broekaert and Johan Martaens started De Sleutel and De Kiem in Belgium, and in Ireland, the Colemine Lodge was established. Don Mario Picci together with Juan Corelli, assisted by Daytop in New York, founded CEIS, Rome.

During the next decade (the 1980s), TCs in Switzerland, Norway, Finland, Spain, Portugal, Poland, and Greece were soon developed. The only country in Europe that seemed immune to the TC "virus" was France. One of the reasons for this might be the strong influence on the French mental health sector of Lacan's psychoanalytic approach that led to the creation of different programs [9].

The Italian TCs—and later the Spanish ones—assisted in the development of the Latin American communities, while in Asia and Australia the first TCs were helped to get started by North American programs such as Daytop in New York. In Africa, there are very few organizations operating that call themselves TCs, and this is a rather recent development.

The International Federations

It didn't take long for national and continental federations to develop among these diverse programs. The first federation to be created was that of the North American TCs.

Treatment Communities of America (TCA)

It was founded in 1975 as a nonprofit member-led professional association in the United States and Canada. It was originally called Therapeutic Communities of America, but in 2011 its board of directors approved a name change of the association to Treatment Communities of America (keeping, thus, the same initials). It was a move that was met with a lot of controversy; some thought that TC core values were being diluted. The board of directors, though, believed that the name change more accurately reflected the complexity and diversity of the services provided by the member organizations. Today, TCA is a federation of over 600 programs that provide a variety of integrated services which include, among others, preventive care, education and assessment, detoxification, residential and nonresidential treatment, family therapy, mental health services, and vocational and housing assistance. These services target many different groups, including army veterans. TCA also recognizes the importance of advocacy and of networking with lawmakers, policymakers, and other stakeholders. To that extent, TCA produces a weekly newsletter that provides its members with "Public Policy Updates" and also hosts a monthly "Public Policy" conference call.

European Federation of Therapeutic Communities (EFTC)

After 4 years of intensive deliberation, the constitution of EFTC was formally signed in Dusseldorf, Germany, on the 6th of February 1981. As one reads in the EFTC site,

> this formal meeting in Dusseldorf was, in many ways, the first stage of an odyssey to secure our dream of a network of drug treatment communities across Europe, learning from each other and delivering recovery-oriented services through peer support and mentoring, challenging negative behavior and role modeling: what we call community as method.

With more than 70 member organizations from 27 countries and associate members from Israel, Lebanon, Iran, Colombia, United States, and Japan, the EFTC is one of Europe's largest and oldest recovery networks. Some years ago, a few member programs withdrew their membership in disagreement with the federation's direction and formed a new smaller organization, the EURO-TC. Recently, the two bodies are organizing together common events and are discussing about conjoint projects. Organizations that belong to EFTC run prison TCs, community-based TCs, day programs, and street-based services, among other things. Members are also active contributors to the International Journal of Therapeutic Communities, and the federation manages an online discussion forum, the only such forum available anywhere in the world. EFTC is also closely linked with the European Working Group on Drugs Oriented Research (EWODOR), the oldest European research network dealing with substance use disorders [18]. Also, EFTC has run, so far, 16 biennial international conferences.

Australasian Therapeutic Communities Association (ATCA)

The ATCA, together with TCA, are the most homogenous federations since they are comprised of two countries (Australia and New Zealand; United States and Canada). They are also the two associations that have an executive director. Following a special premier's conference in Melbourne that brought together treatment providers from across Australia, TC leaders met again the following year (1986) and established the Australian (later to become the Australasian) Therapeutic Communities Association. Today, ATCA members manage more than 70 TCs in community and custodial settings across Australia and New Zealand (Fig. 7.2).

Member organizations provide, among others, services for detoxification, family therapy, gambling addiction treatment, mental health counseling, and child care facilities.

Notably, the association puts a very strong emphasis on research, having established partnerships with the universities of New South Wales, Monash, Newcastle, Deakin, Wollongong, Adelaide, and Curtin. In 2014, it also produced the ATCA Standard for Therapeutic Communities and Residential Rehabilitation Services which was certified by the Joint Accreditation System of Australia and New Zealand (JAS-ANZ).

Federación Latinoamericana de Comunidades Terapéuticas (FLACT)

The Latin American Federation of Therapeutic Communities (FLACT) was established in Campinas, Brazil, in 1986 as a regional group of the World Federation of Therapeutic Communities (WFTC). The main goal of FLACT is to consolidate the national associations members, strengthen their training programs, and create permanent links among them. FLACT has members in 23 countries. What is rather unique with the Latin American Federation is that in many South American states, strong national federations exist: the Brazilian Federation of Therapeutic Communities (FEBRACT), the Colombian Federation

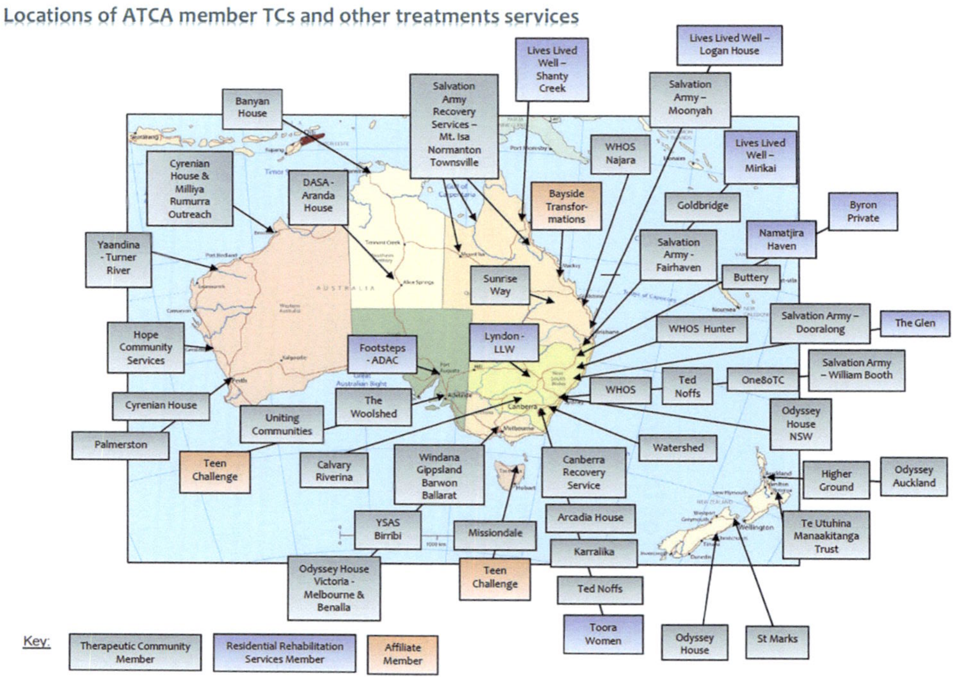

Fig. 7.2 TCs in Australasia (www.atca.com.au)

Therapeutic Communities (FECCOT), the Mexican Federation of Therapeutic Communities (FEMEXCOT), and the Peruvian Association of Therapeutic Communities (PTCA). These four national bodies together with Argentina they have 285 therapeutic communities. FLACT focuses strongly on staff training, and its biennial Latin American Conference of Therapeutic Communities (CLACT) is attended by thousands of professionals.

Federation of Therapeutic Communities in Asia (FTCA)

The Asian is the newest addition to the international TC federation roster. During the World Federation of Therapeutic Communities (WFTC) board meeting held in Bangkok in November 2017, the WFTC executive council withdrew its recognition of the Asian Federation of Therapeutic Communities as it has been inactive for 4 years. Four organizations from Indonesia, the Philippines, India, and Sri Lanka were assigned with the task to start anew. They met in Manila twice, and in November of 2018 at the 27th WFTC Conference in Bangkok, Thailand, the new Federation of Therapeutic Communities in Asia was established. The mission of the FTCA is:

> to establish and support Therapeutic Communities that will serve as havens for people who have fallen prey to all manners of addiction as well as those who have behavioral disorders. Together with their families they can help each other regain hope and rebuild their lives as they live in a healing community free of substance and non-substance dependencies and interacting freely based on universal values and principles.

The FTCA uniquely adds a fourth dimension, the spiritual, to their biopsychosocial approach described in their vision statement. In 2019, FTCA plans to inaugurate its International Institute of Therapeutic Communities (IITC) in the Philippines, a joint effort by two of its member organizations, SELF from the Philippines and Kasih Mulia Foundation (KMF) from Indonesia. This vibrant young organization already has 36 members and strives for a larger membership since there are many TCs in the region (in Iran, for example, where George De Leon's book *Therapeutic Community as Method* has been translated and widely used, there is a great number of TCs).

The World Federation of Therapeutic Communities (WFTC) and the Declaration of Mallorca

The WFTC was established in 1980. It is the forum where all the regional/continental federations come together. For many years, and with the financial assistance of the US State Department, the WFTC was led by Daytop founder Monsignor William B. O'Brien, a Catholic Cardinal from New York. After O'Brien's death and the merger of Daytop with Samaritan Village in 2015, the organization took a different turn. The contributions of all the regional federations increased, and in two meetings, first in Genoa, Italy (2010), and then in Mallorca, Spain (2016), two declarations were produced.

In December 2016, a group of about 150 experts on therapeutic communities from 26 countries gathered at the city of Palma de Mallorca and formulated the Declaration of Mallorca, a document intended to provide a 10-year action plan for improving TC services and interventions worldwide. After a long and intense deliberative process, the text that was unanimously accepted by all participants describes best where therapeutic communities from around the world stand today. The following is a summary of the declaration's main themes:

- Target groups: TC interventions have to be adapted to the participants' needs and their cultural, economic, social, and religious diversity. There should be an emphasis given to specific vulnerable groups and to the fight against stigmatization. Also, the gender perspective into the treatment of addictions must be a constant consideration of the services provided.
- Social reintegration: TCs welcome aftercare services focused on improving the social reintegration of the participants.

Families and other social networks are key factors in reducing relapse.

- Research: the importance of vigorous research and evidence-based outcomes is emphasized. TCs are encouraged to be involved in publishing scientific papers and to collaborate with academia and the research community.
- Finances: the WFTC acknowledges that transparency and accountability are fundamental aspects of the functioning of organizations in the addiction field. TCs should also produce cost-benefit studies to demonstrate the value of the TC model to the various stakeholders.
- Staff: the need for continuous and external supervision of the staff is of paramount importance. TCs require the presence of interdisciplinary professional teams, including experts by experience. TC leadership must be inspirational, transparent, and of service to the community.
- Communication and advocacy: in order to increase society's awareness about the harmful consequences of addiction, communication through the Internet and social media is crucial. The WFTC's strategic plan also requires a strong and continuous presence of the TC movement at international fora, in collaboration with the regional federations and other civil society networks.

In March of 2017, the Declaration of Mallorca was presented and accepted as an official document at the 56th Session of the Commission on Narcotic Drugs (CND) in Vienna.

A Case Study: KETHEA in Greece

Perhaps the best way to illustrate the current status of TCs around the world is to present the Greek organization KETHEA (Therapy Center for Dependent Individuals). The Greek situation concerning substance use disorders is unique, mainly for two reasons. First, all services provided are free of charge. This includes prevention, harm reduction, various treatments (including medication-assisted treatment), rehabilitation, family therapy services, etc. Second, the therapeutic community approach was the first to be introduced in the country, at least 10 years before the first state methadone clinic came into existence. Another important recent development is the financial impact of the economic recession, leading individuals to use cheaper substances, such as *shisha* (a combination of methamphetamine and other toxic additive chemicals) and heroin (the main drug of choice). This is the KETHEA story.

1980s: Early Beginnings

In the early seventies, throughout Europe, the developments in social psychiatry were radical. In France and Italy, new philosophical paradigms and the civil rights movement give birth to antipsychiatry and deinstitutionalization [17]. Amidst a subsequent economic recession, the widespread of individuals with mental health disorders and significant substance use out of warehousing institutions and into the community led to growing popular disappointment in these reforms. The "open doors" policy of the psychiatric establishments was increasingly considered good willed but romantic [5].

In Greece, the situation was different. After World War II, the country suffered a 4-year civil turmoil and then, from 1967 to 1974, a military dictatorship. As a result, the Greek state was suspicious of any new ideas that seemed to challenge the status quo. Because welfare was also underdeveloped, the traditional extended family filled in the gap in the system of care. Given that there were no services designed for individuals with addiction, drug users would end up in psychiatric hospitals or prison.

Greek psychiatry, having an institutionalized and biological orientation, became synonymous with neurology [1]. The first university departments of psychology and sociology were established only after 1982.

With the first officially declared deaths by drugs in 1980, the problem of substance use and addiction received national attention and took a central position in the general political discussion about public health.

In 1981, Greece became a full member of the European Union. In October of the same year, the Socialist Party was elected to govern for the first time in modern Greek history. Its main election campaign slogan was "change." Within this new political and social atmosphere, significant changes took place in the welfare and health system. In the context of these changes and due to the increasing phenomenon of drug use and abuse among younger populations, in 1983 the Ministry of Health entrusted a psychiatrist with the task of organizing and setting up treatment facilities for drug addicts in Greece.

The psychiatrist, Phoebus Zafiridis, completed his doctorate in Switzerland and had some experience of drug abuse treatment. Following a formative visit to the Dutch TCs, he suggested to the Greek Ministry of Health that they should create a similar multiphase program to combat the drug abuse problem.

In August 1983, the counseling and detoxification centers started their operation, and 3 months later on the 27th of November, ITHACA, the first TC in Greece, was created. ITHACA was founded as a part of this specialized program near the city of Thessaloniki.

The fundamental philosophic principle of ITHACA was that the drug problem is mainly a social problem that relates to the given social structure and familial interpersonal relationships. Addiction is not regarded as simply an illness in the psychiatric or medical sense of the term, but as a complex biopsychosocial problem. Consequently, treatment cannot be undertaken unless the participation is voluntary and drug-free.

The name ITHACA, a symbolic name, is today a household word in Greek society. Ithaca is the island where Ulysses, a hero of the Trojan War, originated. In modern Greek literature and more specifically in Cavafy's poem Ithaca, the name symbolizes the journey home.

During this early period, the Greek government was supportive, as the development of a specialized treatment program for drug users was one of its priorities. Although its function was not understood, the therapeutic community was representing a new direction which was in agreement with the general atmosphere of change.

ITHACA operated as a pilot program during the first 4 years (1983–1987) and it belonged to the National Welfare Organization. This status changed drastically with the law 1729/1987, when ITHACA becomes a nongovernmental organization, the Therapy Center for Dependent Individuals (KETHEA).

1990s: Transition Time

In the early nineties, the public health agenda in Greece was dominated by the fear of widespread HIV infection and AIDS. Also in this decade, the portrayal of substance use on Greek private television networks led to the perception of an epidemic.

In 1993, the Greek parliament passed a law that promulgates the establishment of a governmental organization, OKANA. OKANA was presented as a new solution to the drug addiction problem in Greece. The policy was to promote methadone programs, at the expense of the established drug-free programs. Before, TCs were the panacea; now, panacea was medication-assisted treatment and harm reduction.

During this period, KETHEA started to focus on the collection of data and the training of professionals, as the need for evaluating the effectiveness of treatment programs became more obvious.

While the reorganization was difficult, KETHEA adopted new schemes and differentiated its approach, in order to respond to the growing treatment needs of a broader spectrum of drug users, with the help of research and practice. Changes included democratic procedures to discuss the policy and the goals of the organization, decentralization of decision-making and the therapeutic programs, and emphasis on parallel supervision and evaluation, both internal and external. Furthermore, the aim was to increase the number as well as the size of therapeutic interventions and to improve the services offered. Every program was given the opportunity to organize its own intervention, relevant to geographic location, unique relationships with the local community, available human resources, and, most importantly, the special needs of the people to whom it was addressed. A critical dimension of continuous training and education in new methods was introduced. KETHEA also started to examine and assess its services in connection with the population: were they attractive and relevant? As a result of these studies, KETHEA began to provide new services for drug using populations that had not approached its facilities before.

Entering the Twenty-First Century: Development and Integration

The successful effort of KETHEA to adapt to the new external conditions and the ever-changing needs of individuals with substance use disorders, through internal restructuring and the launching of new services, led the organization into new paths of development.

Having realized that not all individuals with substance use disorders are the same and that there is a need for adopting different models for different population groups, KETHEA designed and implemented new services such as treatment programs for ethnic minorities, addicted mothers and their children, an emergency telephone helpline, support centers for discharged prisoners, harm-reduction activities, and crisis intervention centers. The organization now runs counseling centers and TCs in 20 prisons nationwide and provides services to people who are addicted to alcohol, gambling, and the Internet. It has a prevention, a research, and an education department (the latter cooperates with outside institutions, such as the University of California in San Diego and the Aristotle University of Thessaloniki).

KETHEA's external supervisors include George DeLeon, David Deitch, Martien Kooyman, Thomas Maclellan, Giles Amado, and Demetrius Iatridis, among others.

In 2001, the National School of Public Health developed an outcome study of KETHEA, demonstrating the effectiveness of its model. The study involved persons enrolled in KETHEA Therapeutic Communities in 1994–1995. Looking at this sample of individuals at least 5 years after they entered treatment, the study showed that of those who had completed 1 year of treatment:

- 67.7% had abstained from the use of any illegal substance.
- 72.7% had avoided any legal trouble (arrests, convictions, imprisonment, etc.).
- 83.7% were in employment.

Even those who had participated in a therapeutic community for less than a year (but for at least 90 days) derived many benefits from their participation. These benefits include a general improvement in their health, lower levels of HIV/AIDS and hepatitis C, a reduced likelihood of involvement in illegal activities, and improved social and interpersonal ties (Fig. 7.3).

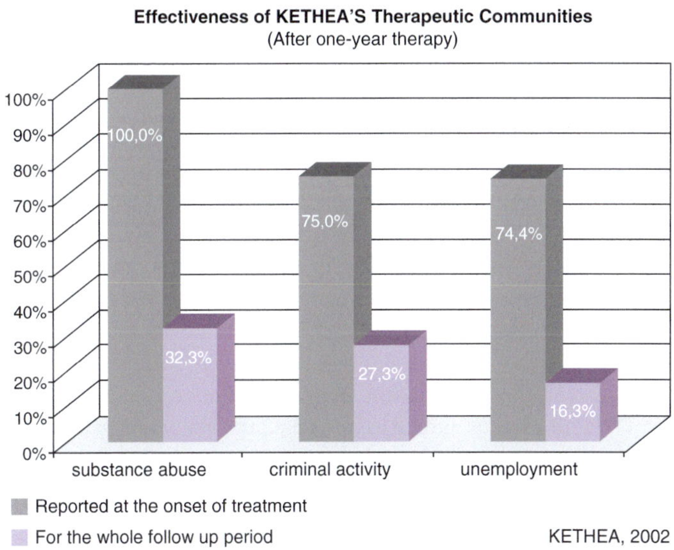

Fig. 7.3 National School of Public Health Research (2001)

KETHEA is also a special consultant to the Economic and Social Council (ECOSOC) of the United Nations and with over 110 units across the country is considered one of the largest solid organizations of its kind in Europe.

The model of the therapeutic community is still used by KETHEA, but it has also evolved its theory and practice to combine self-help, solidarity, active participation, shared responsibility, democracy, and permissiveness concepts. A distinctive characteristic of this new phase in KETHEA's history is the way in which its relationship with the governmental organization OKANA has progressed from a competitive interaction to a fruitful collaboration and exchange of ideas [16].

Since Greece is facing the most difficult economic and social crisis of its modern history, the challenge for an NGO like KETHEA is a crucial one. With almost no new hirings since 2006, with less government funding (overall reduction between 2009 and 2019 is approximately 33%), and with more people in need seeking the services offered, the organization has to rediscover in itself, once more, relevant and effective treatment.

Recent TC Research

Although therapeutic communities are one of the most common and most widely available treatment models in the world, scientific evidence demonstrating their effectiveness is still limited. This is partly due to the variety of approaches implemented within the framework of the TC model and also because of the difficulty to develop study designs to measure its effectiveness and efficacy.

In 2018, the Association Proyecto Hombre in Spain and KETHEA in Greece agreed to initiate a pilot study aimed at investigating the interplay between certain dimensions of vulnerability on the severity of addiction [2]. In this collaboration they found a willing partner in the Prevention, Treatment and Rehabilitation Section of the United Nations Office on Drugs and Crime

(UNODC). PH too is a nongovernmental organization in special consultative status with the United Nations Economic and Social Council (ECOSOC). Since 1984, Proyecto Hombre provided services for over 35,000 people with substance use disorders and their families with more than 220 facilities across Spain.

The main hypothesis of the study is that there is a determining relationship between family history of substance use; co-occurring mental health disorders; history of emotional, physical, or sexual abuse; and the severity of drug dependence. The instrument that was used was the EuropASI which is the European version of the 5th edition of ASI (Addiction Severity Index) developed in the United States by McLellan in 1990. The ASI was initially created in 1980 at the University of Pennsylvania [14] with the aim of providing a clinical evaluation of patients with substance use disorders. ASI allows for a multidimensional diagnosis of addiction problems, assessing their severity in a biopsychosocial context.

The sample consisted of 201 cases, and the persons who took part had undergone a treatment program in KETHEA's and Proyecto Hombre's TCs in 2017. EuropASI's dual interviewing modalities were administrated to all cases, i.e., at the beginning of treatment and after completion of the program, as a follow-up. A sociodemographic analysis was carried out by country of origin, gender, age, academic degree, marital status, months in prison, and employment situation (Figs. 7.4–7.10).

A further analysis was carried out concerning the perception of substance use as the main problem. Findings showed some differences in the samples, including more alcohol and cocaine use in the Spanish group and more heroin or polysubstance use in the Greek group (Figs. 7.11 and 7.12).

The preliminary results of this analysis, which is still underway, show that the subjects have experienced substantial improvements in their quality of life (Fig. 7.13).

In the years to come, the ultimate goal of this research is to include a global representativeness; TC programs in other regions of the world are expected to join.

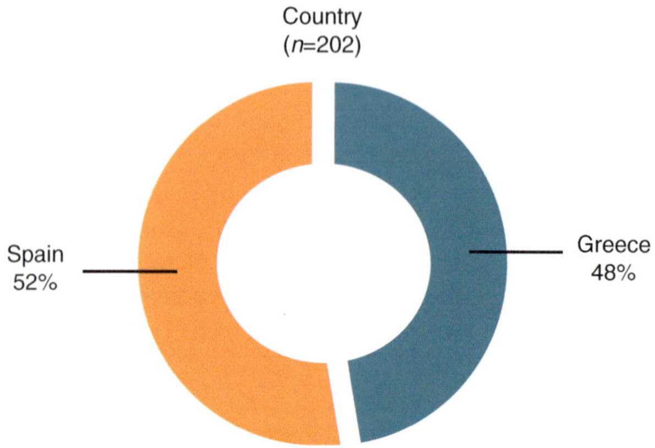

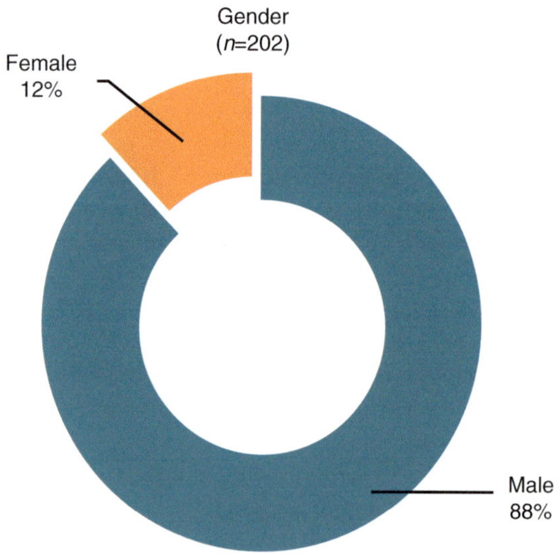

Figs. 7.4–7.10 Sociodemographic information

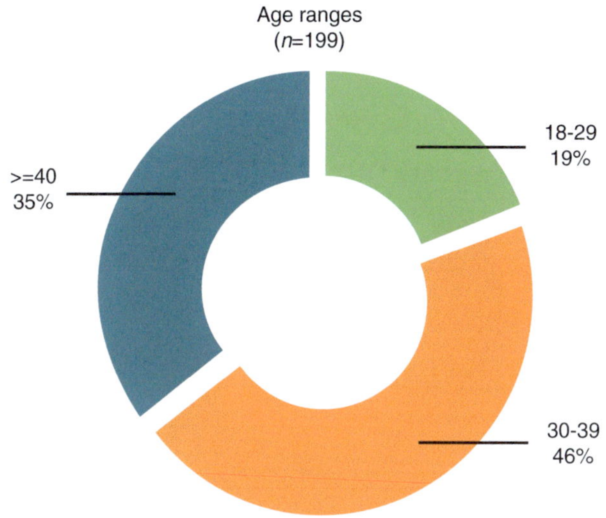

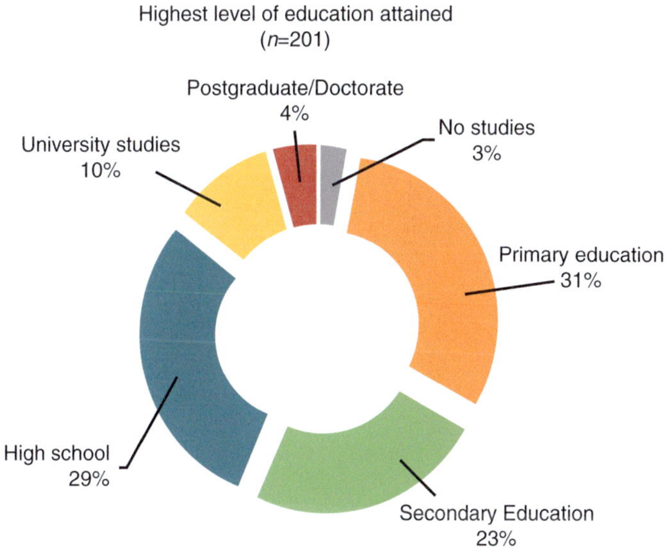

Figs. 7.4–7.10 (continued)

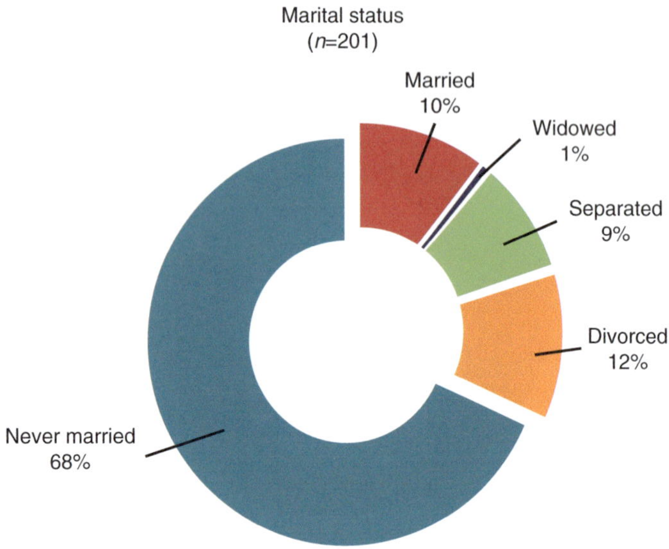

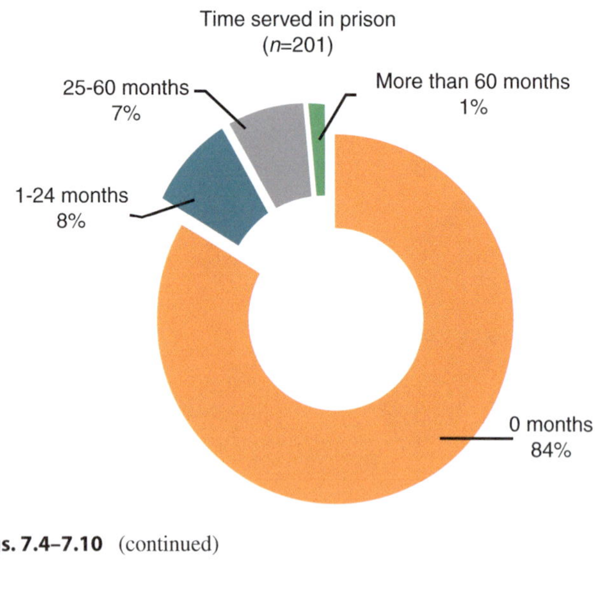

Figs. 7.4–7.10 (continued)

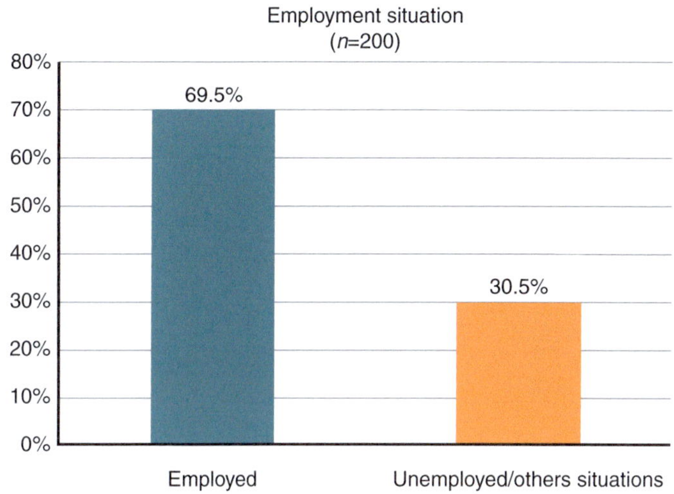

Figure 7.4–7.10 (continued)

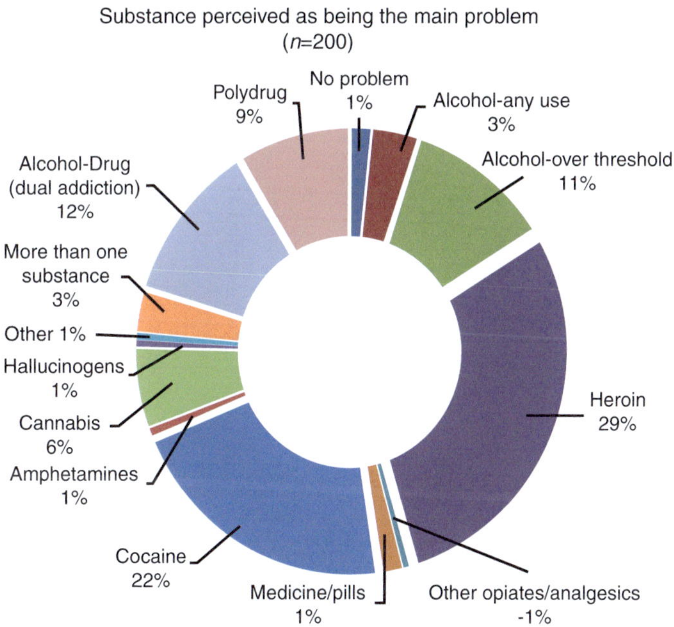

Figs. 7.11 and 7.12 Substance use

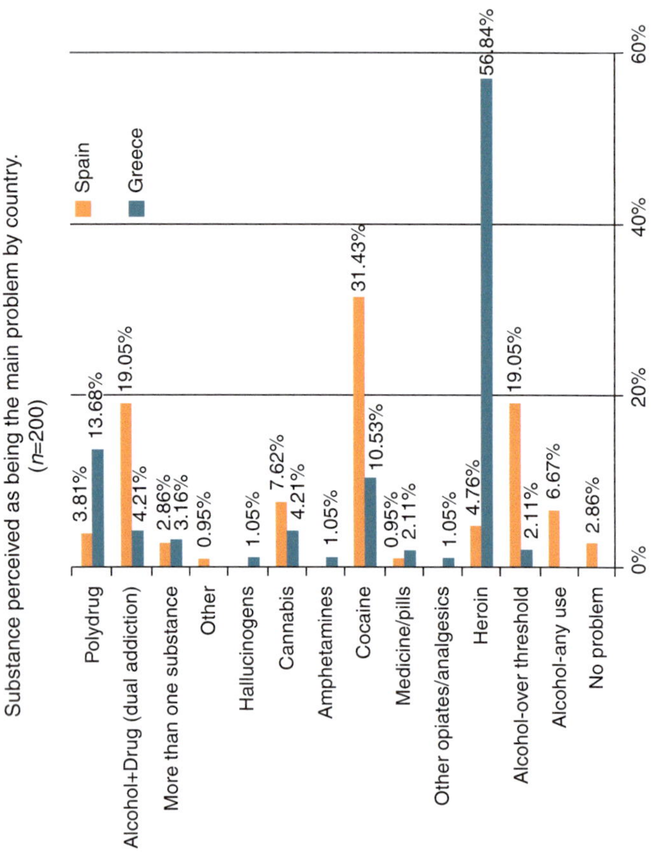

Figs. 7.11 and 7.12 (continued)

A quick view			
200 patients undergoing a treatment programme at Kethea and PH in 2017 entered the study The male/female ration in both programmes was 9/1 2/3 of them were aged less than 40 years and 1/5 less than 29	The substance perceived as most problematic was different between Kethea and PH patients (Greek patients reporting heroin or polydrug use and Spanish patients reporting cocaine, alcohol and alcohol/other drugs) Significantly long history of substance use in all patients (between a and 11 years) with onset use between 14 and 17 years depending of substance	The majority of patients (90% of sample) had no history of previous treatments. About 1/5 of patients had history of previous arrests	The EUROPASI domain scores of the 200 patients were ranked as follows (from most to least affected) - Family/social relationships: 5.84 points out of a range from 0-9 - Psychiatric (perhaps best described as symptoms rather than status): 4.97 points out of a range from 0-9 - Employment support status: 4.33 points out of a range from 0-9 - Alcohol use related status: 3.92 points out of a range from 0-9 - Medical status: 2.97 points out of a range from 0-9 - Legal status: 2.65 points out of a range from 0-9 Despite differences in drug of choice profiles, the EUROPASI score per domin did not vary significantly between Greek and Spanish samples

Fig. 7.13 Preliminary results

Conclusion

Therapeutic communities have developed significantly since their inception. Today, TCs operate all over the world, providing services to diverse groups of people with substance use disorders. In view of the current opioid epidemic in North America, the model of the therapeutic community may serve as an important additional treatment approach that is uniquely adaptable to local contexts and able to flexibly incorporate other modalities of treatment. Further, there is an opportunity to contribute novel research to the growing body of evidence demonstrating the effectiveness of the TC model.

The word "therapon" (therapist) is first recorded in Homer's Iliad. It originally signified the servant who helps a warrior put on his armor before battle. Health providers, and more specifically addiction professionals, are exactly this: therapists, servants who serve people in their need. They equip vulnerable individuals so that they can go fight their personal battles. As the Declaration of Mallorca concludes: "This declaration reaffirms the commitment of the Therapeutic Community movement to serve addicted populations and their social networks all over the world by restoring their hope, dignity and personal well-being."

References

1. Blue A. The creation of Greek psychiatry Athens. Athens: Exantas; 1999.
2. Bonet X, Kafentzaki V, Koutsoukou A, Mullor J, Papanastasatos G, Rueda F. Relation between family history of substance use, co-occurring mental health disorders, history of emotional, physical or sexual abuse and adversities and treatment responses and outcome. Association Proyecto Hombre and KETHEA Bulletin; 2019.
3. Bridger H. The development of the Northfield experiment. Bull Menn Clin. 1946;10:71.
4. Bunt GC, Muehlbach B, Moed CO. The Therapeutic Community: international perspective. Subst Abus. 2008;29:81–7.
5. Clark DH. The therapeutic community. Br J Psychiatry. 1977;131:553–64.
6. Deitch DA. The treatment of drug abuse in the therapeutic community: historical influences, current consideration, future outlook. In: Drug Use in America: Problem in Perspective: Second Report, vol. 4, Washington: Commission on Marihuana and Drug Abuse; 1973. p. 158–75.

7. DeLeon G, Rosenthal MS. Therapeutic communities. In: DuPont R, Goldsstein A, O'Donnell PJ, editors. Handbook on drug abuse; 1979. p. 39–48.
8. Freudenberger HJ. The Therapeutic Community revisited. Am J Drug Alcohol Abuse. 1976;3(1):33–43.
9. Gerstein DR, Harwood H. Treating drug abuse: a study of the evolution, effectiveness and financing of public and private drug treatment systems, vol. 1. Washington: National Academy Press; 1990.
10. Jones M. The therapeutic community: a new treatment method in psychiatry. New York: Basic Books; 1953.
11. Kennard D. An introduction to therapeutic communities. London: Rutledge and Kegan Paul; 1983.
12. Kooyman M. The therapeutic community for addicts: intimacy, parent involvement and treatment outcome. Amsterdam: Swets and Zeittinger; 1993.
13. Main T. The hospital as therapeutic institution. Bull Menn Clin. 1946;10:66.
14. McLellan AT, Kushner H, Metzger D, et al. The fifth edition of the addiction severity index. J Subst Abuse Treat. 1992;9(3):199–213.
15. Poulopoulos C. An interview with Harold Bridger. EFTC Newsl. 1997;6:10–1.
16. Poulopoulos C. Dependencies: the Therapeutic Communities. Athens: Greek Letters; 2005.
17. Roth M, Kroll J. The reality of mental illness. New York: Cambridge Press; 1986.
18. Vanderplasschen W, Vandevelde S, Broekaert E. Therapeutic communities for treating addictions in Europe: evidence, current practices and future challenges. Luxemburg: Publications Office of the European Union; 2014.
19. Yablonsky L. The therapeutic community. New York City: Gardner Press; 1989.

Therapeutic Communities and the Judicial System in the United States

8

Andrew Tuck and Lauren Stossel

Introduction

Substance use disorders (SUDs) are a widespread issue among incarcerated people in the United States. The prevalence of substance use disorders in prisons is five times higher than in the general population, as more than half of prison inmates in the United States meet DSM-IV criteria for a substance use disorder [6, 8]. This phenomenon partly relates to the association between addiction and criminal behavior.

The "War on Drugs" was a large contributing factor to the high rates of SUDs in prison populations. The War on Drugs was a large campaign of policies instituted in the 1970s to curtail illegal drug use in the United States. It included increased penalties for drug offenses, such as mandatory minimums of up to 15 years for drug possession and sales. It also introduced significant sentencing disparities between powder and crack cocaine, leading [1] to widely

A. Tuck (✉)
Columbia University Vagelos College of Physicians & Surgeons, New York, NY, USA
e-mail: andrew.tuck@columbia.edu

L. Stossel
Correctional Health Services, NYC Health+Hospitals, New York, NY, USA
e-mail: lstossel@nychhc.org

J. D. Avery, K. A. Kast (eds.), *The Opioid Epidemic and the Therapeutic Community Model*, https://doi.org/10.1007/978-3-030-26273-0_8

disproportionate incarceration of African Americans and those of low socioeconomic status [5, 34]. In the 1970s, drug offenses accounted for 10% of new prison admissions; by the late 1980s, they accounted for up to 35% of admissions [3]. The War on Drugs has significantly strengthened the relationship between imprisonment and substance use in the US prison population. While crack cocaine initially drove the increased rates of incarceration, the opioid epidemic in the United States has recently captured attention for the burden it places on the correctional system: in one recent study, about 20% of those with prescription opioid use disorder and about 40% of those with past-year heroin use reported recent involvement with the criminal justice system, compared to less than 3% in the general population [57].

The association between substance use and incarceration also extends to the relationship between addiction and criminogenic behavior. Nearly one-fifth of United States prison inmates report obtaining money for drugs as a motive in their offense, and about one-third were intoxicated at the time of their offense [8, 33]. In one study in the United States, more than half of inmates self-reported use of illicit substances during their imprisonment [42].

Because of the high prevalence of addiction in the prison population, and because of the association of substance use disorders with both initial crime and recidivism, successful management of substance use in the corrections system is of tremendous importance. While drug education, group-based counseling, and individualized counseling have all been studied and implemented for treatment of SUDs in incarcerated populations, no single treatment modality has clearly prevailed over the others in terms of uptake, and all are commonly used to some extent [46].

One treatment option that has experienced relatively broad uptake in the correctional setting is the therapeutic community. The therapeutic community is a group-oriented self-help approach to addiction treatment. Patients live together in self-sustaining communities, often with counselors who are in recovery from addiction themselves. Therapeutic communities emphasize a holistic approach to recovery from substance use, including an emphasis on rebuilding social skills and developing prosocial values as a means to create lasting recovery from substance use [9].

In the United States, one of the most common settings for therapeutic communities is the correctional system, specifically prisons. (TCs are much less common in jails because they require longitudinal involvement [6]). TCs are particularly well suited to prisons for a number of reasons. First, the approach to addiction implicit in the therapeutic community model—that addiction is a "social" disease and is best corrected by the development of prosocial skills and values [9]—matches the rehabilitative goal of the correctional system. Compared to other forms of drug treatment, the holistic and community-oriented approach of the therapeutic community may be especially beneficial to a population struggling to succeed or survive safely in the larger community. Second, in addition to an implicit focus on developing personal responsibility and fostering prosocial behaviors, therapeutic communities have traditionally focused on practical goals, such as stable housing and obtaining sustainable employment. Such an approach is particularly valuable to the prison population, who often experience limited social prospects on release. Third, incarcerated users are ensured housing, which is typically one of the most significant expenses of therapeutic communities [54]. Last, it is generally agreed that longer durations of stay produce better outcomes. Benefits of TC participation may not be seen before 90 days of involvement are completed [40], and a typical prison TC program lasts between 6 and 12 months [21]. In the United States, the average prison sentence length is just over 5 years, allowing the majority of prisoners to have ample time to participate [7]. For these reasons therapeutic communities offer a compelling method of treatment of substance use disorders in incarcerated populations.

History of Therapeutic Communities and the Judicial System

Therapeutic communities in the United States began in the 1950s and spread to the American correctional system shortly thereafter. The earliest prison TCs, such as Asklepieion in Illinois or the Federal Correctional Institution therapeutic community in Oxford,

Wisconsin, enjoyed initial successes. Corrections administrators were eager to reduce recidivism and relapse in prisoners, and inmates were eager to take advantage of benefits offered by early TCs. These benefits included favorable impressions to parole boards, access to the higher-quality housing reserved for participants, and the ability to speak frankly to other inmates and even prison staff (as the therapeutic community concept encourages) [56]. This initial popularity was somewhat curtailed by a backlash among corrections researchers calling into question the evidence base behind the most common substance use treatment programs used in prisons, including therapeutic communities [39]. The tempered enthusiasm among policy makers and laypeople temporarily decelerated the expansion of residential treatment-based programs in the United States. However, in the late 1980s, when the War on Drugs began to rapidly crowd prisons with substantial numbers of offenders with substance use problems, interest in finding a scalable and effective modality for addiction treatment was revitalized [53].

A new wave of outcomes research on prison-based therapeutic communities, such as Stay'n Out in New York and Cornerstone in Oregon, debuted in the context of this revitalization. Stay'n Out was a NIDA-funded study and one of the earliest randomized controlled trials of prison TCs. Results from this study found that the rearrest rate of males who participated in the TC was significantly lower than both the no-treatment control and those who participated in either counseling or a milieu group [55]. Similar results were found for females. In addition to these encouraging findings on recidivism, the Stay'n Out study was influential insofar as it helped establish an optimum minimum time in treatment as nine to twelve months [53]. In Oregon, the Cornerstone program, though not a randomized controlled trial, found similarly encouraging results for reducing recidivism [13]. Additionally, research from this program may have bolstered enthusiasm for the holistic approach of the TC, as they found improvements across several measures of psychological well-being in addition to reduced recidivism [12].

The initial successes reported by these programs restoked interest in therapeutic communities as a potential modality for substance use treatment in the corrections system. Consequently, with the passage of the Violent Crime Control and Law Enforcement Act of 1994 [50], substantial federal funds were allotted to the development of residential substance abuse treatment (RSAT) in prisons. RSAT grants led to rapid creation of residential treatment programs. About a quarter of these were traditional therapeutic communities with nearly 60% combining elements of therapeutic communities with other treatment modalities (e.g. 12-step groups) [21]. As of 2003, there were more than 2000 RSAT programs spread across all 50 states [35]. The promising successes of these prison TCs increased funding for more TC development and provided opportunities for further research [53].

Profile of Therapeutic Communities in Prison

Prison TCs serve a wide range of prisoners in both general and specialized (i.e., for substance use treatment) detention centers and have been used for inmates of both sexes over a variety of age groups [21]. Although prison TCs are a distinct entity from TCs in the general community, the foundational principles are generally the same. Participants live, work, and sleep in the same place (albeit due to the confines of a prison). In some programs (about a fifth [46]), participants live together in a segregated unit to better embody the communality emphasized in the TC approach. However, not all prison TCs can completely segregate their members from the wider prison population. In accordance with the community-based TC model, prison TCs characterize addiction as a deficit of social adjustment necessitating character development on the part of the participant. Participants are required to engage in self-reflection and self-evaluation to develop an ethic of personal responsibility and social accountability. The TC expects participants to adjust their attitudes and values to fit societal expectations. Participants work to correct motivations and behaviors that might lead to relapse and develop skills and abilities seemingly unrelated to addiction, but viewed as necessary to function in society. Such skills include conflict resolution and timely completion of chores.

Historically, prison TCs have been ideologically split. One approach, originating in the United States, emphasizes gradual and merit-based progression through a hierarchy. The other, originating in Britain, emphasizes a more democratic approach. Modern prison TCs commonly have elements of both [49]. Participants may receive weekly educational seminars on relevant topics in psychology, addiction, and philosophy. Daily group meetings and frequent communal events are a backbone of prison TCs. Participants are encouraged to engage in candid discussion about their own shortcomings and to "call out" other participants and staff on their behavior [45]. Like community TCs, prison TCs involve a culture of encouragement and mutual support, as well as confrontation. Participants are continually challenged to reflect on the effects of their actions on others, but are also rewarded with increased trust and authority (as well as perks like more desirable chores) within the TC.

Some factors that differentiate prison TCs from TCs in the general community stem from funding limitations or changes, involvement of prison administrators, high rates of staffing changes, and other infrastructural limitations inherent to a prison setting. Additionally, the primary goal of prisons is security, not treatment, and thus security will override the treatment goals of the TC when the two are felt to be at odds [53]. Similarly, the daily scheduling of the prison will trump over the programming of the TC, meaning that participants in prison TCs may spend fewer hours per day in treatment than participants in general TCs. Additionally, in community TCs, many staff are in recovery or even graduates of TCs themselves. However, at many prisons, hiring policies pose barriers to taking on staff with histories of arrest or substance abuse, thus limiting both the diversity and number of staff in an already understaffed setting [21].

One of the most notable distinctions between the pure TC model that exists in the community and the iteration of TCs developed for incarcerated populations is the blending of other treatment modalities with the therapeutic community. Because substance use treatment within prisons is government sponsored, prison TCs may be subject to pressures and incentives not present in TCs in the general community. Among programs receiving federal RSAT funding, only about one-quarter were pure TCs. Most programs merged elements of TCs with other modalities, such as cognitive-behavioral therapy or 12-step groups [21]. The inclusion of other modalities may differentiate prison TCs from each other and from TCs in the general community, making comparisons difficult.

Efficacy of Prison TCs

Several systematic reviews and meta-analyses have investigated the efficacy of prison TCs. One of the earliest meta-analyses, by Pearson and Lipton, analyzed studies between 1968 and 1996 to assess the efficacy of three prison drug treatment programs (boot camps, group counseling, and TCs) for reducing recidivism. These three programs were compared a treatment-as-usual comparison group who received generic group counseling for recidivism that was not focused on substance use [36]. Of the 20 studies that met inclusion criteria, 7 focused on TCs. The authors found that TCs were the only one of these modalities that produced significant reductions in recidivism compared to treatment as usual (Table 8.1).

Aos et al. examined the literature published between 1970 and 2005 on drug treatment programs for patients involved in the correctional system [2]. Of the 92 evaluations found, thirteen examined the efficacy of TCs in prison (six with aftercare, seven without) (Table 8.1). The authors found that participation in prison TCs was associated with a 5.3% decrease in recidivism compared to offenders receiving no treatment. Offenders receiving aftercare in addition to prison TC treatment demonstrated a modest further benefit for a total of a 6.9% reduction in recidivism. For comparison, cognitive-behavioral therapy, the other major modality for prison drug treatment investigated in this study, was associated with a 6.8% decrease in recidivism after release. Relapse was not examined.

In one of the largest and most recent meta-analyses, the authors used 74 evaluations published from 1980 to 2011 [31]. Four different types of prison-based drug treatment programs

Table 8.1 Meta-analyses of drug treatment programs in prisons that included therapeutic communities

Meta-analysis	Studies included	Main interventions examined	Outcomes examined	Results	Summary
[2]	92 published evaluations (1970–2005) of drug treatment programs for adult offenders involved in correctional system, 21 of which focused on prisons	Prison TCs with aftercare ($n = 6$) Prison TCs without aftercare ($n = 7$) Cognitive-behavioral drug treatment in prison ($n = 8$)	Recidivism	TCs with aftercare: 6.9% reduction in recidivism (compared to treatment as usual; $p < .001$) TCs without aftercare: 5.3% reduction in recidivism ($p = .001$), cognitive-behavioral treatment: 6.8% reduction in recidivism ($p < .001$)	Prison TCs were effective in reducing recidivism. They were more effective than cognitive-behavioral drug treatment, but only when paired with aftercare

[31]	74 evaluations published between 1980 and 2011 examining effects of prison drug programs for juveniles and adults	TCs ($n = 35$) Boot camps ($n = 2$) Medication-assisted treatment (MAT; $n = 6$) Counseling-based programs ($n = 26$)	Recidivism and relapse	*Recidivism reduction (odds ratio, [95% confidence interval]):* TCs (1.40, [1.14, 1.71]), boot camp (1.10, [0.48, 2.50]), MAT (0.57, [0.34, 0.95]), counseling (1.53, [1.20, 1.94]) *Relapse reduction (odds ratio, [95% confidence interval]):* TCs (1.33, [0.92, 1.93]), boot camp (0.56, [0.16, 2.01]), MAT (2.10, [1.03, 4.27]) counseling (0.77, [0.35, 1.70])	For relapse, MAT was most effective, followed by in-prison TCs. For recidivism, counseling was most effective, followed closely by TCs Overall, TCs were most consistent in reducing *both* outcome variables
[36]	30 published and unpublished studies between 1968 and 1996 on drug programs for imprisoned offenders, both adult and juvenile	TCs ($n = 7$) Boot camps ($n = 6$) Drug-based group counseling ($n = 7$)	Recidivism	Therapeutic communities (weighted mean $r = .13$ $p = .25$) Boot camps (weighted mean $r = .05$; $p = .163$) Group counseling (weighted mean $r = .04$, $p = .054$)	TCs were effective in reducing recidivism. Boot camps and drug-based group counseling were not

(medication-assisted treatment, boot camps, counseling, and therapeutic communities) were compared. Both relapse and recidivism were examined. The authors found that, on average, these programs reduced relapse after release by 15%. (Table 8.1) The most effective program for reducing relapse was medication-assisted therapy by far, followed by TCs. The other two program types, including counseling, were not found to lower drug relapse. For recidivism, counseling was found to be the most effective. The other two treatment types, medication-assisted treatment and boot camps, were not found to be effective for reducing recidivism. The authors concluded that, while other treatment types outperformed prison TCs for relapse and recidivism considered individually, it was the most consistently effective treatment type for reducing both, across a wide range of offenders.

Despite the promising findings of systematic reviews and meta-analyses on this topic, a number of methodological flaws and limitations have been noted in the current literature on prison TCs. Many systematic reviews and meta-analyses note that studies on prison TCs rarely meet the highest level of quality; rigorous experimental design is rare [32]. Some limitations are inherent to TCs themselves. For example, blinding participants is virtually impossible [43]. Some analyses have noted the presence of publication bias in favor of prison TC treatment [31]. Randomization errors are common [43], as are concerns about self-selection and attrition bias [6]. Notably, in analyses that only consider the most rigorous studies or control for selection bias, prison TCs still appear to have robust effects on recidivism and relapse [31, 37].

While research on prison TCs has demonstrated that they are one of the most consistent interventions in reducing both recidivism and relapse, their benefits may extend beyond these outcomes. For example, the Cornerstone TC in Oregon showed a significant improvement in participants' self-esteem and a decrease in symptoms like depression, hopelessness, and feelings of social incompetence [12]. A systematic review examining psychological outcomes in addition to relapse and recidivism found that many studies on TCs evidenced substantial decreases in psychopathological symptoms like anxiety and distress in their participants [47]. Post-release employment is another valuable outcome to consider, especially as it is correlated with relapse and recidivism [52]. A study of the Amity TC in California found that those who completed treatment at both a prison TC and an aftercare TC had significantly higher rates of employment at follow-up compared to the control group (this effect was only present for those who completed aftercare) [38]. This is consistent with literature on community-based TCs demonstrating improved employment prospects after participation [41]. However, the effects of prison TC participation on post-release employment are generally under-researched [52].

Cost-Effectiveness

Although the literature on the cost-effectiveness of TCs in the community is limited [43], most studies generally suggest that they are a cost-effective form of treatment (i.e., the costs of the program are outweighed by the funds saved by reduction in crime) [14, 15, 58]. Prison TCs differ from community TCs in several ways that may impact cost-effectiveness. On one hand, prison TCs deal with a population that is traditionally considered difficult to treat. On the other, prison-based drug treatment programs in general tend to be more cost-effective than their community counterparts [10], because they directly target a population that is most at risk for future crime. While TCs are a relatively expensive form of drug treatment overall [48], TCs in prison are less so, as the primary expense of TCs—housing—is covered by the prison [54].

Overall, the available empirical evidence suggests that TCs are cost-effective. One of the earliest studies to examine the cost-effectiveness of modern prison TCs was the New Vision program in Kyle, Texas [19]. This analysis yielded two important findings. First, treatment of inmates at high risk for recidivism was much more cost-effective than treatment of inmates at lower risk. The authors concluded that the marginal decreases in recidivism for inmates already at low risk were small enough that less intensive (and less expensive) modalities might be more cost-effective. Second, the TC was only cost-effective for inmates who also completed aftercare [19].

The latter finding is consistent with a subsequent study that examined the CREST program in Delaware, which found that TC treatment was only effective when participants completed aftercare [27, 28]. The authors found that, for prisoners who completed a combined TC/work-release program without aftercare, it costed $65 in treatment to prevent one day of reincarceration. This compares to $19 per incarceration-day prevented for those who completed aftercare. A cost-effectiveness analysis of the Amity program in California also found that prison TC treatment was only effective when participants enrolled in aftercare [27–29]. (Of note, in both the CREST and Amity programs, participants were randomly assigned to TC treatment or controls, but volunteered for aftercare. This introduces the possibility of a selection bias that inflates the success of those who completed aftercare.)

Subsequent reviews have generally found prison TCs to be a cost-effective form of drug treatment for imprisoned populations. A 2012 meta-analysis by Drake found TCs to be an effective but expensive method of drug treatment for incarcerated populations, saving $2.59 in prevented crime for every $1 spent on treatment [10]. While effective, prison TCs were less cost-effective than a composite of other drug treatment programs in prison, which yielded an average of $4.79 in savings for every $1 spent. For juvenile offenders treated for substance use while incarcerated or in the community, TCs were more cost-effective than non-TC treatments ($2.47 vs $2.16 saved, per dollar spent on treatment).

Notably, while costs saved by reduction in crime are the most commonly examined outcome in estimating cost-effectiveness, they are not the only one. In one study of a California prison, prisoners involved in TC treatment were less expensive than prisoners not involved in treatment. The difference was primarily driven by lower numbers of in-prison disciplinary actions, inmate complaints, and lockdowns due to behavioral issues [59]. Thus, in addition to the costs saved by society, prison administrators may benefit from incorporating TCs into their prisons.

Opioid Use Treatment in Correctional Settings

While one benefit of therapeutic communities is their applicability to a wide variety of addictive substances, the landscape of illicit drug use in the United States is increasingly shifting toward opioids. Thus, it is worth examining TCs in the corrections system specifically as a treatment for opioid use disorder, especially given the close connection between illicit opioid use and criminal activity [57].

Compared to other substance use disorders, one fortunate element in treating opioid use disorder is the existence of a robust pharmacological treatment: opioid replacement therapy. Opioid replacement therapy, or the administration of long-acting opioid agonists (e.g., buprenorphine and methadone) to patients addicted to heroin or short-acting prescription opioids (e.g., oxycodone), is backed by a wide range of research spanning decades. This research has consistently shown that opioid replacement therapy reduces relapse compared to counseling-based treatment alone [17, 31] and is generally considered the gold standard for the treatment of opioid use disorder [23–26]. Large reviews also indicate that opioid replacement therapy reduces recidivism among incarcerated patients [11, 22].

Despite the evidence supporting the superiority of medication-assisted treatment compared to counseling-only approaches, a number of factors limit the uptake of opioid replacement therapy in the correctional setting. These include state and local regulations [16], unawareness of the evidence for opioid replacement therapy, concerns about diversion of medications, and the misperception that opioid replacement therapy just "replaces one addiction with another" [30, 51]. Consequently, opioid replacement therapy is significantly underutilized in correctional settings [6]. In one study of 50 correctional agencies (e.g., prisons, jails, drug courts), 83% of jails and prisons offered some form of opioid replacement therapy. However, this was almost entirely restricted to pregnant women and acute detoxification and, to a lesser extent, continuation of outpatient therapy [16]. For example, only one of the twelve prisons examined offered methadone initiation to prisoners not already on methadone treatment.

Of the 15 factors surveyed by Friedmann and co-investigators, the second most popular reason endorsed for opposing opioid substitution therapy was that the prison preferred drug-free treatment options (security concerns were first). The third was that opioid substitution therapy was felt to be "inconsistent with the agency's treatment philosophy" [16]. Thus, despite the strong evidence behind methadone and buprenorphine, prisons demonstrate an institutional bias toward non-pharmacologic treatment.

One such treatment, of course, is the therapeutic community. However, very few studies of TC efficacy speak to opioid use disorder specifically. It is therefore not clear whether participants with opioid use disorder fare better or worse, on average, than other TC participants, or how they differ qualitatively.

Similarly, few studies comparing opioid substitution therapy to residential treatment programs exist. Such studies face a number of barriers, including participants' lack of willingness to participate in the arm of the study not involving treatment with methadone [20, 25]. One early study comparing TCs to methadone maintenance therapy found that long-term TC participants outperformed patients who received methadone on a number of measures, including drug use and rearrest [4]; however, the study was later criticized for flaws in its randomization process [43].

Comparing opioid substitution-based treatments with TCs, however, suggests a false dichotomy, as TCs and opioid substitution therapy are not mutually exclusive modalities. Historically speaking, the philosophy of therapeutic communities has emphasized drug-free living, with abstinence as the ultimate goal [9]. TCs in the community rarely accept patients taking methadone or buprenorphine, and those that do typically do so only temporarily for the purposes of detoxification. Patients on opioid substitution therapy can be perceived as a threat to group unity by staff or other TC participants, or as using a "crutch" to remain off illicit drugs [18].

While the therapeutic community philosophy has traditionally been at odds with opioid substitution-based approaches, it has also proven itself to be a very flexible modality. Since their inception, TCs have been adapted to a wide range of populations, including both sexes, juveniles, homeless persons, and drug users with comorbid mental illness [18]. It is conceivable that the incorporation of opioid substitution approaches could be a future adaptation. Some early research has indicated that opioid substitution therapy can be successfully integrated into TCs without compromising outcomes. One "test of equivalency" study compared TC participants on methadone in the community to participants in the same TC not on methadone. Results showed that these two groups did not differ on key outcomes including retention in treatment, alcohol and illicit opioid use, and sexual risk behaviors [44].

Although this study was based on a TC in the community, there is little reason to think that prison TCs would preclude the integration of opioid substitution therapy. In fact, prison TCs seem more likely than community TCs to make pragmatic compromises to the TC philosophy, or to combine modalities. As noted above, only a quarter of residential substance use treatment programs in prisons are pure TCs. The majority involve a combination of TC principles and other therapeutic approaches [21]. Accordingly, while the usual concerns about limited access to opioid substitution therapy still apply, correctional settings may be fertile grounds for new approaches to opioid use disorder that combine TCs with opioid substitution-based approaches.

Conclusions

Prison TCs treat a different population than community TCs and will likely yield different results [47]. Nevertheless, they have a long history of successful use in the American correctional system and are, in many ways, especially well suited to prisons and prisoners. Decades of research on TCs for patients involved the correctional system and, more specifically in prisons, support its use as an efficacious and cost-effective tool to reduce substance use in this vulnerable population. Prison TCs may have several benefits over other forms of drug treatment programs, including evidence that they reduce both recidivism and relapse, where other programs may affect just one or neither [31]. Furthermore, prison TCs may offer broad psychosocial benefits that extend beyond the usual measures of drug use and recidivism.

However, there is much to learn about TCs and their potential to help individuals with substance use disorders. This is especially true in the midst of an opioid epidemic that disproportionately affects individuals involved in the criminal justice system. Methodological limitations in research on prison TCs limit the conclusions that can be drawn from these programs. Furthermore, literature on prison TCs for those who specifically use illicit opioids is almost nonexistent. Despite these challenges, prison TCs have proven to be a pragmatic and flexible approach to solving substance use. These qualities may prove uniquely useful in adapting to a changing landscape of substance use.

References

1. Anti-Drug Abuse Act of 1986, 3207, Pub. L. No. 99-570, 100 Stat. (1986).
2. Aos S, Miller MG, Drake E. Evidence-based adult corrections programs: what works and what does not: Washington State Institute for Public Policy; 2006.
3. Austin J, McVey AD. NCCD prison population forecast, 1989: the impact of the war on drugs. United States of America; 1989.
4. Bale RN, Van Stone WW, Kuldau JM, Engelsing TM, Elashoff RM, Zarcone VP. Therapeutic communities vs methadone maintenance: a prospective controlled study of narcotic addiction treatment: design and one-year follow-up. Arch Gen Psychiatry. 1980;37(2):179–93.
5. Beaver AL. Getting a fix on cocaine sentencing policy: reforming the sentencing scheme of the Anti-Drug Abuse Act of 1986. Fordham L Rev. 2009;78:2531.
6. Belenko S, Hiller M, Hamilton L. Treating substance use disorders in the criminal justice system. Curr Psychiatry Rep. 2013;15(11):414.
7. Bonczar T. State Prison Admissions, 2006: sentence length by offense and admission type. Washington: Bureau of Justice Statistics; 2010.
8. Bronson J, Stroop J, Zimmer S, Berzofsky M. Drug use, dependence, and abuse among state prisoners and jail inmates, 2007–2009. Washington, DC: United States Department of Justice, Office of Juvenile Justice and Delinquency Prevention; 2017.
9. De Leon G. The therapeutic community: theory, model, and method. New York: Springer Publishing Co; 2000.
10. Drake E. Chemical dependency treatment for offenders: a review of the evidence and benefit-cost findings (Document No. 12-12-1201). Olympia: Washington State Institute for Public Policy; 2012.

11. Egli N, Pina M, Skovbo Christensen P, Aebi MF, Killias M. Effects of drug substitution programs on offending among drug-addicts. Campbell Syst Rev. 2009;5(3).
12. Field G. The Cornerstone program: a client outcome study. Fed Probat. 1985;49:50.
13. Field G. The effects of intensive treatment on reducing the criminal recidivism of addicted offenders. Fed Probat. 1989;53:51.
14. French MT, McCollister KE, Sacks S, McKendrick K, De Leon G. Benefit–cost analysis of a modified therapeutic community for mentally ill chemical abusers. Eval Program Plann. 2002;25(2):137–48.
15. French MT, Sacks S, De Leon G, Staines G, McKendrick K. Modified therapeutic community for mentally ill chemical abusers: outcomes and costs. Eval Health Prof. 1999;22(1):60–85.
16. Friedmann PD, Hoskinson R Jr, Gordon M, Schwartz R, Kinlock T, Knight K, et al. Medication-assisted treatment in criminal justice agencies affiliated with the criminal justice-drug abuse treatment studies (CJ-DATS): availability, barriers, and intentions. Subst Abus. 2012;33(1):9–18.
17. Gordon MS, Kinlock TW, Schwartz RP, Fitzgerald TT, O'Grady KE, Vocci FJ. A randomized controlled trial of prison-initiated buprenorphine: prison outcomes and community treatment entry. Drug Alcohol Depend. 2014;142:33–40.
18. Greenberg B, Hall DH, Sorensen JL. Methadone maintenance therapy in residential Therapeutic Conmmunity settings: challenges and promise. J Psychoactive Drugs. 2007;39(3):203–10.
19. Griffith JD, Hiller ML, Knight K, Simpson DD. A cost-effectiveness analysis of in-prison therapeutic community treatment and risk classification. Prison J. 1999;79(3):352–68.
20. Gunne L-M, Grönbladh L. The Swedish methadone maintenance program: a controlled study. Drug Alcohol Depend. 1981;7(3):249–56.
21. Harrison LD, Martin SS. Residential substance abuse treatment for state prisoners: implementation lessons learned. Washington, DC: Office of Justice Programs; 2003.
22. Koehler JA, Humphreys DK, Akoensi TD, Sánchez de Ribera O, Loesel F. A systematic review and meta-analysis on the effects of European drug treatment programmes on reoffending. Psychol Crime Law. 2014;20(6):584–602.
23. Kourounis G, Richards BDW, Kyprianou E, Symeonidou E, Malliori M-M, Samartzis L. Opioid substitution therapy: lowering the treatment thresholds. Drug Alcohol Depend. 2016;161:1–8. https://doi.org/10.1016/j.drugalcdep.2015.12.021.
24. Marsch LA. The efficacy of methadone maintenance interventions in reducing illicit opiate use, HIV risk behavior and criminality: a meta-analysis. Addiction. 1998;93(4):515–32.
25. Mattick RP, Breen C, Kimber J, Davoli M. Methadone maintenance therapy versus no opioid replacement therapy for opioid dependence.

Cochrane Database Syst Rev. 2009;(3) https://doi.org/10.1002/14651858.CD002209.pub2.
26. Mattick RP, Breen C, Kimber J, Davoli M. Buprenorphine maintenance versus placebo or methadone maintenance for opioid dependence. Cochrane Database Syst Rev. 2014;(2) https://doi.org/10.1002/14651858.CD002207.pub4.
27. McCollister KE, French MT, Inciardi JA, Butzin CA, Martin SS, Hooper RM. Post-release substance abuse treatment for criminal offenders: a cost-effectiveness analysis. J Quant Criminol. 2003a;19(4):389–407.
28. McCollister KE, French MT, Prendergast M, Wexler H, Sacks S, Hall E. Is in-prison treatment enough? A cost-effectiveness analysis of prison-based treatment and aftercare services for substance-abusing offenders. Law Policy. 2003b;25(1):63–82. https://doi.org/10.1111/1467-9930.00140.
29. McCollister KE, French MT, Prendergast ML, Hall E, Sacks S. Long-term cost effectiveness of addiction treatment for criminal offenders. Justice Q. 2004;21(3):659–79. https://doi.org/10.1080/07418820400095941.
30. McMillan GP, Lapham SC. Staff perspectives on methadone maintenance therapy (MMT) in a large southwestern jail. Addict Res Theory. 2005;13(1):53–63.
31. Mitchell O, Wilson D, Layton MacKenzie D. The effectiveness of incarceration-based drug treatment on criminal behavior. Campbell Syst Rev. 2012;2012(18).
32. Mitchell O, Wilson DB, MacKenzie DL. Does incarceration-based drug treatment reduce recidivism? A meta-analytic synthesis of the research. J Exp Criminol. 2007;3(4):353–75. https://doi.org/10.1007/s11292-007-9040-2.
33. Mumola CJ, Karberg JC. Drug use and dependence, state and federal prisoners, 2004: US Department of Justice, Office of Justice Programs, Bureau of Justice; 2006.
34. Palamar JJ, Davies S, Ompad DC, Cleland CM, Weitzman M. Powder cocaine and crack use in the United States: an examination of risk for arrest and socioeconomic disparities in use. Drug Alcohol Depend. 2015;149:108–16.
35. Pealer JA. Correctional rehabilitation and Therapeutic Communities: reducing recidivism through behavior change. New York: Taylor & Francis; 2017.
36. Pearson FS, Lipton DS. A meta-analytic review of the effectiveness of corrections-based treatments for drug abuse. Prison J. 1999;79(4):384–410. https://doi.org/10.1177/0032885599079004003.
37. Pelissier B, Wallace S, O'Neil JA, Gaes GG, Camp S, Rhodes W, Saylor W. Federal prison residential drug treatment reduces substance use and arrests after release. Am J Drug Alcohol Abuse. 2001;27(2):315–37.
38. Prendergast ML, Hall EA, Wexler HK, Melnick G, Cao Y. Amity prison-based therapeutic community: 5-year outcomes. Prison J. 2004;84(1):36–60. https://doi.org/10.1177/0032885503262454.

39. Prendergast ML, Wexler HK. Correctional substance abuse treatment programs in California: a historical perspective. Prison J. 2004;84(1):8–35.
40. Sacks S, Chaple M, Sacks JY, McKendrick K, Cleland CM. Randomized trial of a reentry modified therapeutic community for offenders with co-occurring disorders: crime outcomes. J Subst Abus Treat. 2012;42(3):247–59.
41. Sacks S, Sacks JY, McKendrick K, Banks S, Stommel J. Modified TC for MICA offenders: crime outcomes. Behav Sci Law. 2004;22(4):477–501. https://doi.org/10.1002/bsl.599.
42. Simpler AH, Langhinrichsen-Rohling J. Substance use in prison: how much occurs and is it associated with psychopathology? Addict Res Theory. 2005;13(5):503–11. https://doi.org/10.1080/16066350500151739.
43. Smith LA, Gates S, Foxcroft D. Therapeutic communities for substance related disorder. Cochrane Database Syst Rev. 2006;(1):CD005338.
44. Sorensen JL, Andrews S, Delucchi KL, Greenberg B, Guydish J, Masson CL, Shopshire M. Methadone patients in the therapeutic community: a test of equivalency. Drug Alcohol Depend. 2009;100(1–2):100–6.
45. Springer DW, McNeece CA, Arnold EM. Traditional treatment settings and approaches. In: Substance abuse treatment for criminal offenders: an evidence-based guide for practitioners. Washington, DC: American Psychological Association; 2003. p. 113–23.
46. Taxman FS, Perdoni ML, Harrison LD. Drug treatment services for adult offenders: the state of the state. J Subst Abus Treat. 2007;32(3):239–54. https://doi.org/10.1016/j.jsat.2006.12.019.
47. Vanderplasschen W, Colpaert K, Autrique M, Rapp RC, Pearce S, Broekaert E, Vandevelde S. Therapeutic communities for addictions: a review of their effectiveness from a recovery-oriented perspective. Sci World J. 2013;2013:427817.
48. Vanderplasschen W, Vandevelde S, Broekaert E. Therapeutic communities for treating addictions in Europe. Evidence, current practices and future challenges. Luxembourg: Publications Office of the European Union; 2014.
49. Vandevelde S, Broekaert E, Yates R, Kooyman M. The development of the therapeutic community in correctional establishments: a comparative retrospective account of the 'democratic' Maxwell Jones TC and the hierarchical concept-based TC in prison. Int J Soc Psychiatry. 2004;50(1):66–79.
50. Violent Crime Control and Law Enforcement Act of 1994, Pub. L. No. 103–322, 108 Stat.
51. Wakeman SE. Why It's inappropriate not to treat incarcerated patients with opioid agonist therapy. AMA J Ethics. 2017;19(9):922.
52. Welsh WN. A multisite evaluation of prison-based therapeutic community drug treatment. Crim Justice Behav. 2007;34(11):1481–98.

53. Wexler H, Prendergast ML. Therapeutic communities in United States' prisons: effectiveness and challenges. Ther Communities. 2010;31:157.
54. Wexler HK. The success of therapeutic communities for substance abusers in American prisons. J Psychoactive Drugs. 1995;27(1):57–66.
55. Wexler HK, Falkin GP, Lipton DS. Outcome evaluation of a prison therapeutic community for substance abuse treatment. Crim Justice Behav. 1990;17(1):71–92.
56. Wexler HK, Love CT. Therapeutic communities in prison. NIDA Res Monogr. 1994;144:181–208.
57. Winkelman TA, Chang VW, Binswanger IA. Health, polysubstance use, and criminal justice involvement among adults with varying levels of opioid use. JAMA Netw Open. 2018;1(3):e180558. https://doi.org/10.1001/jamanetworkopen.2018.0558.
58. Yates R. Recovery we can afford: an analysis of a sample of comparative, cost-based studies. Ther Communities. 2010;31(2):145.
59. Zhang SX, Roberts RE, McCollister KE. An economic analysis of the in-prison therapeutic community model on prison management costs. J Crim Just. 2009;37(4):388–95.

9 San Patrignano: Lessons from the Italian Experience

Gabriele Manella, Giovanni Pieretti, Alessandra Landi, and Bruno Genetti

An Overview of Addiction Treatment Services and the Official Data on Use in Italy

Drug use trends are complex and ever changing, and supplying data on these is extremely difficult, as is outlining addiction treatment services. We have opted to use data from the Annual Report to the Italian Parliament (carried out by the Department for Anti-Drug Policies) and EMCDDA annual reports (the European Monitoring Center for Drugs and Drug Addiction) to introduce this topic.

Italy's drug addiction treatment system stands out in Europe. The public sector and private services work together and have been strengthened through an accreditation system within the National Health Service that identifies healthcare providers offering services for substance use disorders. This system as a whole has made significant progress in the treatment of heroin and cocaine addictions: drug-related deaths have decreased in recent

G. Manella (✉) · G. Pieretti · A. Landi
Department of Sociology and Business Law, University of Bologna, Bologna, Italy
e-mail: gabriele.manella@unibo.it; giovanni.pieretti@unibo.it; alessandra.landi5@unibo.it

B. Genetti
Centro Studi Explora, Padua, Italy
e-mail: bruno.genetti@centroexplora.it

J. D. Avery, K. A. Kast (eds.), *The Opioid Epidemic and the Therapeutic Community Model*, https://doi.org/10.1007/978-3-030-26273-0_9

years, and the same trend is to be found in acute viral hepatitis, HIV, and AIDS among drug users [2]. However, overdose deaths increased in 2018 (mirroring the American crisis), and heroin use is increasing, with most deaths involving this opioid. The behavioral addictions (gambling, Internet gaming disorder, etc.) also present a new challenge with their increasing recognition.

The Italian treatment system is divided into 638 public services for addictions (*SerD*) and 917 accredited private services (TCs). 21,458 new users were treated by SerD in 2016, and the total number of users was 143,271. Opioid-related cases were the most frequent with 62,868 people, while high-risk opioid user numbers in Italy are estimated to range from 180,000 to 230,000 [3]. Cannabinoids user numbers have also recently increased, as has related morbidity due to a marked increase in the psychoactive constituents (THC) of marijuana products. 11% of SerD users in 2016 were treated for cannabinoids and 12% of hospital admissions were related to this substance. Most SerD patients are male, and their average age ranges from 30 to 54 years. New users are younger than those already in treatment (the average age is 32 vs. 41 years).

Concerning TCs, the DPA data [2] shows that 15,563 people were treated in 2016, and 4764 of these began treatment over the last year.

The Italian Therapeutic Community Model

Italian TCs have developed over the last 40 years and represent a unique and significant therapeutic modality for substance use disorders in the country [7]. Among international organizations focused on addiction treatment and scientific research, the Italian TC model is considered unique. The heterogeneous services and practices across Italian TCs share certain cultural values. Rural Italian culture, incorporating the Christian social tradition and a focus on life's essentials—including a sense of home, work ethic, healthy living, and producing and consuming food in community—has formed the basis of a "culture of the essentials" (*cultura dell'essenzialità*) in Italian TCs that fosters a milieu supportive of sobriety and stable recovery.

Many Italian TCs are based on the "collective management of the crisis of presence" (*gestione collettiva di crisi della presenza*), where the close proximity, or "presence," of a community of others is the central dynamic confronting the individual. Residents face an intensive experience of self-examination and accountability to the community, with the motivation for social acceptance and belonging driving cohesion and behavior change in alignment with community values. "Looking at yourself in others" 24 hours per day, every day, is a highly intensive milieu therapy. The effectiveness of Italian TCs in treating addictive disorders relies on an ability to establish this milieu. Treatment requires developing not only individualized treatment plans but also environmental settings designed to enhance progress toward stable recovery. TCs are places where people feel welcome, meet others committed to recovery, share community resources, form relationships and social skills, and where residents are able to develop a new identity separate from their presenting appearance as "an addict" with its sequelae.

Additionally, Italian TCs provide a medium- to long-term residential approach; they do not offer short-term treatment. Long lengths of stay increase the likelihood of stable recovery, the desired outcome for each TC resident. In addition to work on symptoms (e.g., substance cravings), educational interventions aim at full reintegration of the individual into their family system, social network, and occupational niche.

San Patrignano and Peer Therapy

San Patrignano (SanPa) is a TC founded in 1978 by Vincenzo Muccioli and a group of friends who shared his goals. It is located in Coriano, a town a few miles from Rimini, in north-central Italy. SanPa is Italy's largest TC focusing on substance use disorders with a current census of 1050 guests (and a capacity of up to 1200 people) and 250 employees (we will use the term "guests" for people who spent time in SanPa dealing with addiction problems). It is a 250 hectare private estate in the hills. Most of the land is used for agriculture with some also being used for work and training facilities, common areas (kitchen, dining room, theater, basketball arena), accommodation for guests and staff, and administration offices.

SanPa offers long-term therapy (3–4 years) that is highly individualized. Vincenzo Muccioli wrote that "men are not skittles," stressing the need to respect individuality and carefully adjust therapy to each person's unique characteristics. This means that TCs attempt to respect each individual's needed length of stay, assuming that these are unpredictable and specific to each person. It is important that those experiencing drug addiction problems know that they are not required to fit in with some *ideal type*. There is no yardstick against which their performance is measured. What counts is taking one's own time and doing it one's own way (with the help of the TC, of course).

More than 26,000 people have completed therapeutic programs in SanPa over forty years, and outcomes have frequently been positive and long-lasting [8]. Average recovery program duration is about four years: three years plus one year for "reintegration" (*reinserimento*), a step whose main aim is to enable individuals to acquire the occupational skills they need in the outside world.

Programs are completely free, though guests must support themselves through everyday work in the community and for the community. Vincenzo Muccioli also intended the free service as a model of love, a way of giving altruistically. This helps foster the trust and combat the typical suspicious stance of TC guests, who often feel they have been "betrayed" by everyone. Work at SanPa is also a way of engaging guests, of getting them to participate in a common livelihood, promoting a sense of usefulness and helping put food on the table.

At the beginning of a therapeutic program, new guests are placed in an operative "module" of 30 people, at most. These modules are connected to one of the SanPa's work and training sectors. Guests are put under the supervision of a module manager. The manager works with other educators to choose another guest at a more advanced stage in the program who becomes a new guest's tutor, mentoring them through the first year at SanPa. New guests share a room with their tutor and others (six beds per room, at most). There is also a manager in each room. These are the people with whom the guests share most of their everyday lives at SanPa.

Personal growth takes place via daily exchanges with roommates, colleagues, and sector managers (professional educators). These relationships form the network wherein a guest's strengths and fragilities are worked on daily. Additional responsibilities are gradually assigned to individual guests during the program, both in the work sector and other SanPa activities (including athletics, artistic work, and other cultural endeavors). New guests also tutor other guests over time, a way of restoring a sense of usefulness as well as providing an opportunity to experience new forms of gratification—replacing the illusory satisfactions provided by drugs. This process is a "peer therapy," according to which new guests' tutors are people who have themselves experienced drug addiction and worked through the process of recovery.

SanPa's admission rules require guests to be drug-free. If people are not capable of achieving detoxification on their own, they are put in touch with two clinics working with the community for medically supervised withdrawal. Once admitted, SanPa remains an open community, and visits from guests' relatives are allowed, contacts with schools encouraged, and events and conferences organized for those outside the community.

Occupational training is another central component of the therapeutic program: it allows guests to gain professional skills in one of SanPa's work and training sectors. This is an educational intervention aimed toward full habilitation, where the guest develops skills to live in society productively, respecting others' needs and functioning as autonomous individuals with advanced professional skills. Available work sectors include: livestock, call center, kennels, wine cellar, cheese factory, medical center, chemical lab, plantation farm, communication office, kitchen, decoration lab, forge, carpentry workshop, bakery, graphics, plumbing, electrical work, laundry, warehouse management, maintenance, grocery, hospitality management (reception of new guests, dining room management, and serving tables), dental care, gardening and green areas, pizzeria, restaurant, media director, hairdressing, horse stables, and weaving factory. Guests may learn an occupation within these sectors while contributing to the TC's activities and sustainability. Their work allows SanPa to be financially independent of external contributions, from both guests' families and national or regional funding. The budget comes from commercial revenues produced by guests' work and fund-raising.

What emerges at SanPa is a milieu in which certain human functions and capacities are enhanced for those living there. Guests are given the opportunity to learn how to transform their strengths into life opportunities (this is the definition that Amartya Sen gives to the concept of *human functioning*). They can identify additional skills, without which these functions cannot take place: the skill of "making territory," meaning being able to adjust to the surrounding environment and find needed resources, as well as finding a personal meaning to life. "Making territory" is being able to find a renewed will to live abundantly and experience the pleasure of sharing life with others.

Being in nature is also important, as it provides the chance to develop a harmonious relationship with the environment, respecting and safeguarding it. There is no TC if nature is not safeguarded, if there is no respect for every form of life because all life forms have the same dignity. We will again refer to Vincenzo Muccioli here to clarify this aspect of SanPa that attempts to foster the protection of dignity in guests, their relationships, and environment (authors' translation):

> There are no men born with the vocation of being drug addict. Every man was born marked by two distinctive characteristics: limit and imperfection. If we do not recognize our limited and imperfect nature, if we are not aware of the need for human relations to fill our limits and realize ourselves as men, we waste our life in subjection to an 'ego' that leaves us alone in the difficult times. During these times, the vacuums that are awkwardly disguised by our egoism enjoy our weakness, and they emerge violently.

SanPa Follow-Up Studies

Independent follow-up studies at SanPa were begun in 1992 to understand the health, social functioning, and living conditions of former guests. Since then, multiple scientific studies have focused on SanPa's approach, organization, and outcomes [1, 4–6]. We will consider two of these studies: a follow-up study in 1992–1993 and another in 2004–2005.

The first follow-up study [4] used a complex methodology which included: three pretesting questionnaires at various moments at SanPa, the reconstruction of biographies for 30 guests, and interviews with key informants on the topic of work during the therapeutic program. The final tool was a questionnaire consisting of 92 closed questions and 16 open questions. The target of the study was former guests who had spent at least 14 months at SanPa with 2,300 people meeting this requirement, 1,208 of whom were located and contacted and 711 agreed to participate in the study (58.9%).

A first interesting result was linked to the TC size: the authors suggested that a "city effect" positively affected rehabilitation outcomes. Many former guests perceived SanPa as a complex system with its own rules and habits which cannot be changed easily nor radically—more a city than a community. This complexity, which approximates a real-world culture and social setting, is hypothesized to better help guests cope with the inevitable difficulties experienced on their return to society outside the community. Another key element was the importance attributed to work for the purposes of recovering personal dignity. Many former guests stressed that group cohesion was what stood out at SanPa: work was a "moral fact," a means to an end. Sharing with others and self-fulfillment are sequentially connected at SanPa: the former makes the latter possible.

In the second follow-up [6], some of the questionnaire recruitment rules and research tools changed. Only former guests who had stayed at SanPa for at least 36 months were considered. However, those leaving without SanPa's consent were also included in the sample. A further innovation (the first in Italy) was a retention-in-treatment study and follow-up using a combination of sociological and toxicological tools: a questionnaire and the use of hair analysis to detect substance use over the previous five months. A total of 511 former guests were contacted, and reliable information was found on 287 of these. Nearly, 72% were drug-free 2–4 years after the end of the therapeutic program, rising to 78% among those who completed treatment with SanPa's consent.

Retention in treatment was 66% after one year of the program, 53% after two years, and 45% after three years. This is a relatively high rate if we consider that 37% treatment retention at 12 months in methadone programs is considered high by international standards, and the best TCs achieve 35%.

The sociological part of the study consisted of a face-to-face questionnaire. A remarkably wide range of employment was reported by those participating in the study (135 different jobs); this variety was considered a clear indicator of the match between SanPa vocational training and the labor market.

Rates of stable drug-free recovery were also notable. Of 252 participants, 97 had been drug addicted for more than 11 years when they entered SanPa (and some for much longer); follow-up showed that 60% were still alive, in good health, and drug-free. A further sociological outcome was a relatively high level of autonomy: 66% of participants no longer lived with their parents (a high rate in Italy), and 115 had their own families, in most cases with children. Most former guests lived far away from the SanPa community, with their own families and their own jobs. Of course, this does not mean that they are not grateful to the TC that welcomed them at a difficult moment and contributed to getting them through it. Such feelings are often expressed in answers to the questionnaire.

The study ends with findings related to relapse rates for former guests. Firstly, failures are more frequent among former guests who left without SanPa's agreement: 37% as compared to 17.6% of those who ended their programs with SanPa's approval. Gender is another key variable: women relapse less frequently (11.5% vs. 22% of men). Length of stay is also an important factor. Longer length of stay leads to a lower relapse rate: 28% in those spending 36–47 months here, 16% of those who spent 48–59 months, and 11% of those who spent 60 months or more here (the latter, of course, had decided of their own accord to stay longer than the established program). Finally, contact with the context of origin, especially family and neighborhood, was found to be a risk factor for poorer outcome; the relapse rate is significantly higher among those who returned to live in the place they lived in before treatment and among those who returned to live with their families.

The Community Outcome Project

We will conclude by discussing the ambitious Community Outcome project, which provides further evidence for the effectiveness of SanPa's TC model in treating substance use disorders.

Objectives

The focus of the study is therapeutic effectiveness (not theoretical efficacy), with additional assessment of potential moderators, including clinical conditions present at the beginning of the program (severity index), treatment processes, and TC characteristics. The three main assessment areas were:

1. Admission methods (selection criteria, number of applications received vs. number of people accepted, severity index on admission, type of substance detected in toxicological tests)
2. Treatment/rehabilitation in the TC (variations in severity index during treatment, length of stay, dropout rate, time to dropout, dropout reasons, training and professional skills acquired, life skills)
3. Posttreatment/rehabilitation (toxicological tests through hair analysis 12 months after leaving the TC, together with assessments of the quality of life and degree of social and labor market reintegration)

Measurement Tools and Functions

Another aim of the Community Outcome study is to create interdisciplinary tools encompassing the TC's characteristics and user paths, from first contact to program end as far as possible. The study includes seven compilation tools:

1. Short severity index: this is filled in at the beginning of the study to assess individual clinical situation at the start of the TC program.

2. User output service: to assess services provided to users throughout their programs and filled in progressively during the SanPa TC program.
3. Internal outcome monitoring for users: to collect users' information on substance use, attitude toward therapies, aggression levels, participation in community life, project-building skills, and handling of family relations and any relapses (completed progressively during the SanPa TC program).
4. Operator life skills: completed every 6 months during the TC program by users' tutors to compile personal evaluations of skills acquired.
5. User life skills: completed every 6 months by users to compile personal evaluations of perceived life skills acquired.
6. Operator customer satisfaction: completed every 6 months during the TC program by tutors to record user satisfaction, perceptions of their stay, and the services provided.
7. User customer satisfaction: completed every 6 months during the TC program by users to record user satisfaction, perceptions of their stay, and the services provided.

The Community Outcome protocol also includes a drug-free state follow-up, tested via toxicological tools (hair analysis) twelve months after users have left the TC. Written consent for this test is signed by users when they leave SanPa.

Analysis Methods

Preliminary descriptive analysis has been done for some tools (short severity index, life skills for users and operators, customer satisfaction for users and operators). Descriptive profiles were generated after this step via cross-tables with variables from other tools (internal outcome monitoring for users, user output service). The results were used for a multivariate analysis to compare respondent characteristics across the various aspects of the study. The information was also analyzed to generate user life skills and customer satisfaction profiles in relation to the condition at the beginning of the TC program (short severity index).

All statistical analysis used SPSS (version 18) and R software to generate descriptive indexes and tables. Graphs were elaborated with Microsoft Office Excel. Scores on each tool were standardized to a 1–100 scale to make comparative analysis possible. The following normalization formula was used:

$$\frac{\text{Total score} - \text{minimum value}}{\text{maximum value} - \text{minimum value}} \times 100$$

Appropriate statistical tests were applied to more accurately assess association/correlation with the variables studied.

Results

As regards user admission scores (short severity index), a medium–low severity profile was found. This confirmed that SanPa staff admission criteria had been achieved. The area with the highest severity score (58.9, where the maximum possible was 100) was toxicology, while the average severity profile in other areas (medical, social, psychological-psychiatric, and previous treatments) did not exceed 30 out of 100.

Higher severity profile user analysis pointed to greater social problems for foreigners, those with medium-to-low education, those separated or divorced, and people with separated parents. Higher toxicology severity scores were found for younger users, unmarried, and those with no children. Higher medical severity scores were associated with drug type and use method.

It is interesting to note that multivariate analysis (Table 9.1) designed to find users with homogenous internal characteristics highlighted the presence of only two groups, confirming the overall homogeneity of users at the time of admission. The distinctive feature of the two groups is the presence or absence of children, especially underage children. The childless group is relatively younger and includes more single people without stable employment and with higher severity scores in the toxicological and psychological-psychiatric areas. The second group is relatively older, with more married or cohabiting people with lower toxicological

Table 9.1 Cluster analysis results

Variables	Importance	Group 1 *N* = 202 (83.5%)	Group 2 *N* = 40 (16.5%)
Children	1	No (100.0%)	Yes (100%)
Presence of young children (minors)	0.97	No (100.0%)	Yes (97.5%)
Marital status	0.48	Unmarried (95.5%)	Married/ cohabiting (45.0%)
Children living elsewhere and/or in care to social services	0.46	No (100.0%)	No (50.0%)
Children living in same house and/or not in care to social services	0.44	No (100.0%)	No (52.5%)
Age	0.13	27.36	34.53
Toxicology score	0.07	61.55	52.5
Education	0.03	Lower secondary school (61.9%)	Lower secondary school (50.0%)
Social area score	0.02	21.16	24.08
Medical area score	0.02	12.9	16.17
Presence of children	0.01	Natural (96.0%)	Natural (100.0%)
Occupation	0.01	Not stable (53.0%)	Stable (57.5%)
Psychological-psychiatric area score	0.01	25.51	22.62
Primary drug used	0.01	Heroin (60.4%)	Heroin (52.5%)
Parental status	0.01	Together (55.9%)	Together (60.0%)
Gender	0	Male (81.2%)	Male (85.0%)
Presence of father	0	Yes (85.6%)	Yes (82.5%)
Nationality	0	Italian (88.1%)	Italian (92.5%)
Previous treatment area score	0	26.79	27.36
Primary drug taking method	0	Inhaling/per os (58.4%)	Inhaling/per os (57.5%)
Presence of mother	0	Yes (97.5%)	Yes (97.5%)

severity and higher social and medical severity, also due to difficulties caring for their children. A medium-high level of education is common to both groups.

These results were confirmed through further analysis to assess the characteristics of the "less severe" and "more severe" groups for each area of the short severity index. A less severe toxicology score was associated with the presence of children, especially underage children, who lived in the same house and were not in care. This is probably connected to a sense of parental responsibility.

A less severe medical profile emerged for users with a "softer" toxicological profile (where inhalation was the main method of drug taking, for example) and users who did not have separated parents. A less severe social profile emerged in users in stable employment and users who grew up with both parents. On the other hand, a higher tendency to repeat treatments has been found in users who inject opioids.

After analysis on the severity index profiles, further analysis was done on life skills and customer satisfaction throughout the TC program. In particular, comparative analysis was used to assess any differences in user and operator perceptions. The results show significant life skills improvements during the TC program in all the areas considered (mental and physical health, emotions and relationships, training and employment) and in particular in mental and physical health cognitive skills.

A further result emerged from a comparison between user and operator points of view: the former tend to give lower scores than the latter. It is notable, however, that the longer the stay at SanPa, the lower the difference between the two points of view. In many cases, after three years on the TC program, scores assigned by users and operators tend to coincide.

One of the research questions was the length of TC program required for significant life skills improvements. As regards physical and mental health, emotions and relationships, from 6 to 12 months, were observed in both life skills assessment tools (users and operators). Significant improvement in behavior (communicating effectively, management of daily tasks, respect for ethical values, caring for others) requires 6–12 months for users but a

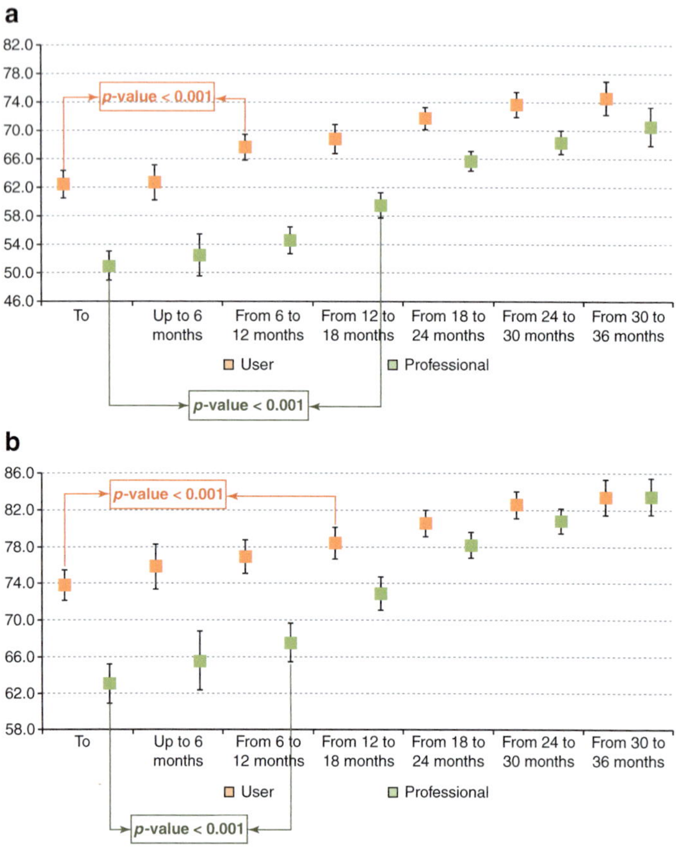

Fig. 9.1 Trends in average life skills scores regarding behavior (**a**) and training and employment (**b**), as reported by users and operators

longer time frame (12–18 months) for operators (Fig. 9.1a). On the other hand, a significant improvement in training and employment skills was perceived after 6–12 months by operators and after 12–18 months by users (Fig. 9.1b).

Regarding dropouts (leaving the TC program before its conclusion), at the time of our study, 61 users out of 233 had left treatment (26.2%). In other words, the retention factor was very high among SanPa guests who participated in the Community Outcome study. 30% of dropouts occurred in the first two months of the TC program and a further 36% in the third or fourth month. Only 20% dropped out after the first year (12 out of 61). Those who dropped out were relatively older (32.1 on average vs. 28.4 years of age among non-dropouts). We also observed that dropout affects opioids and stimulant addicts equally, and those with underage children were at greater risk. We also assessed for a relationship between dropout results with short severity index scores: no significant differences emerged, with slightly higher severity rates in medical, social, and psychological-psychiatric areas.

Conclusion

While it is challenging to study drug addiction treatment comprehensively, this chapter has outlined the efforts made to understand what works in SanPa's TC model. Retention in treatment is high for SanPa across multiple studies. Further, the Community Outcome participants' high retention rates create a strong cohort dataset for further follow-up assessment. Treatment retention increases the population of those engaged in treatment who may reach treatment goals, including full reintegration into society and the labor market, as well as stable recovery from substance use.

References

1. Baraldi G, Piazzi G. La Comunità capovolta: bambini a San Patrignano. Milan: FrancoAngeli; 1998.
2. Dpa - Dipartimento Politiche Antidroga. Relazione annuale al Parlamento 2017 sullo stato delle tossicodipendenze in Italia. Rome: Presidenza del Consiglio dei Ministri; 2017.
3. EMCDDA. 2018 European drug report. Lisbon: European Monitoring Centre for Drugs and Drug Addiction; 2018.
4. Guidicini P, Pieretti G. San Patrignano between Community and Society: a research on the biographic routes of 711 former guests. Milan: FrancoAngeli; 1994.
5. Guidicini P, Pieretti G. San Patrignano: terapia ambientale ed effetto città. Studio sui percorsi di vita degli ospiti della comunità. Milan: FrancoAngeli; 1996.

6. Manfré G, Piazzi G, Polettini A. Beyond the community: multidisciplinary study of retention in treatment and follow-up on former residents of San Patrignano. Milan: FrancoAngeli; 2005.
7. Pieretti G. Per un modello italiano delle comunità terapeutiche. In: Pieretti G, Bovi S, Bottura N, editors. Comunità terapeutica e comunità locale: dalla vulnerabilità alla condivisione. Milan: FrancoAngeli; 2016. p. 33–47.
8. Patrignano S. Un anno di noi: numeri, energia, passioni. Il bilancio di missione. Coriano: Comunità di San Patrignano; 2017.

Index

A
A118G polymorphism, 81
Abstinence-based model, 3
Abstinence-based recovery, 4
ACE, *see* Adverse Childhood Experiences
Acute viral hepatitis, 134
Addiction, 3
  behavioral, 134
  correctional setting, 114–115
  in prisons, 113
  treatment, 3
    resistant in, 76–78
    services, 133–134
  workforce, 25–26
    ex-addict paraprofessionals, 25
    staff burnout, 39
Addiction Severity Index (ASI), 103
Adverse Childhood Experiences (ACE), 38
African Americans, 114
AIDS, 134
Alcohol, 78
Alcoholics Anonymous, 3
Alpha House, 89
American Fix, 19
American Pain Society, 52
American Society of Addiction Medicine's (ASAM), 70
Analogous synergistic effect, 80
Anesthesia-assisted detoxification, 65
"Anti-psychiatry" movement, US, 3
Anxiety, 38
Anxiety-spectrum, 78
ASI, *see* Addiction Severity Index
Australasian Therapeutic Communities Association (ATCA), 92

B
Benzodiazepines, 64
Bion's theory, 80
Bipolar disorder, 38
Boy's Republic, 88
Brazilian Federation of Therapeutic Communities (FEBRACT), 92
Bridger, H., 87
Buprenorphine, 17, 64, 65, 67–69, 75, 77, 125

C
Cancer Pain Monograph, 52
Cannabinoids, 134
Cannabis, 78
CARA, *see* Comprehensive Addiction and Recovery Act

J. D. Avery, K. A. Kast (eds.), *The Opioid Epidemic and the Therapeutic Community Model*, https://doi.org/10.1007/978-3-030-26273-0

Carbamazepine, 66
Cardiac arrhythmias, 67
CBT, *see* Cognitive behavioral therapy
CEIS, Rome, 89
Chemical abuse, 10
Cimetidine, 67
Ciprofloxacin, 67
Clonidine, 64, 69
CND, *see* Commission on Narcotic Drugs
Cocaine, 26, 78, 133
Cognitive behavioral therapy (CBT), 10, 16, 70
Cold turkey, 64
Colemine Lodge, 89
Colombian Federation of Therapeutic Communities (FECCOT), 92–94
Commission on Narcotic Drugs (CND), 96
Community-based TC agencies, 10
Community Outcome project, 141–147
Comprehensive Addiction and Recovery Act (CARA), 2
Corticotropin-releasing hormone (CRH), 69
Crack superseded heroin, 26
CREST program, 124
CRH, *see* Corticotropin-releasing hormone
CYP450, 66

D

Daytop, 89
The Declaration of Mallorca, 96
Deconstructing the Therapeutic Community, 36
Dederich, C., 88
Democratic therapeutic community, 24
Depression, 38
De Sleutel and De Kiem, 89
Detoxification, 63–65
Diacetylmorphine, 51
Dreser, H., 51
Drug abuse research, 102–103
Drug Addiction Treatment Action (DATA), 2000, 68, 72
DSM-IV, 113

E

Economic and Social Council (ECOSOC), 103
Erythromycin, 67
Europe, 49
European Federation of Therapeutic Communities (EFTC), 91
European Monitoring Center for Drugs and Drug Addiction (EMCDDA), 133
European Working Group on Drugs Oriented Research (EWODOR), 91
Evidenced-informed psychosocial treatment, 10
Ex-addict paraprofessionals, 25

F

Federación Latinoamericana de Comunidades Terapéuticas (FLACT), 92–94
Federation of Therapeutic Communities in Asia (FTCA), 94–96
Fentanyl, 27, 57, 58
Fluconazole, 67
Fluvoxamine, 67

H

HAART medications, 66
Harrison Narcotic Act, 1914, 51
Health Parity and Addiction Equity Act, 2008, 72
Hepatitis B, 57
Hepatitis C, 57

Heroin, 51, 55–57, 69, 133
Human immunodeficiency virus (HIV), 1–2, 57, 134
Hybridization, TC, 35–37

I
Inside the Opioid Addiction Crisis, 19
International Federations, 90
International Institute of Therapeutic Communities (IITC), 94
Italian therapeutic community model, 134–135

J
Joint Accreditation System of Australia and New Zealand (JAS-ANZ), 92
Judicial system, 115–117

K
Kasih Mulia Foundation (KMF), 94
KETHEA, 96–102

L
Lacan's psychoanalytic approach, 90
Latin American Conference of Therapeutic Communities (CLACT), 94
Latin American Federation of Therapeutic Communities (FLACT), 92
Length of stay (LOS), 2–4, 71

M
Medication-assisted treatment (MAT), 2–4, 17–19, 65, 70, 75, 80
Medically supervised withdrawal, 63
MET, *see* Motivational enhancement
Methadone, 17, 64–68, 75, 125, 126
Methadone maintenance therapy, 3
Methadone to abstinence (M-A) model, 18
Mexican Federation of Therapeutic Communities (FEMEXCOT), 94
Morphine, 50, 51, 57
Motivational enhancement (MET), 16
Motivational incentives, 37
Motivational interviewing, 10
Mu-receptor opioid agonist, 67
Mutual self-help approach, 16

N
Naloxone, 67, 77
Naltrexone, 65, 68–69, 75, 77
Narcotic addiction, 25
Neurobiological syndrome, 76
N-methyl-D-aspartic acid (NMDA), 69

O
O'Brien, Monsignor William B., 95
Obstetrics, 2
Office-based treatment, 65, 67
"Old school" TC approach, 38
Opioid
  for cancer, 52
  potential alternatives, 57–58
  prescription in pain management, 53–54
  related deaths, 45
  in United States, 46–49
Opioid antagonist maintenance therapy, 64
Opioid detoxification, 64
Opioid epidemic, 1–3, 17–19, 46–49
Opioid receptor agonist, 70
Opioid replacement therapy, 125

Opioids, 45, 64
efficiency in pain management, 54–55
heroin, 55–57
pain management, 49–53
treatment in correctional settings, 125–127
Opioid substitution therapy, 126
Opioid use disorder (OUD), 1, 63, 75, 77
antagonist maintenance therapy, 64
buprenorphine, 67–68
in correctional settings, 125–127
destigmatizing medication-assisted treatment, 65
detoxification, 64–65
heroin, 69
immunotherapies, 70
maintenance treatment, 64–65
methadone, 66–67
naltrexone, 68–69
treatment for, 64–65, 76–78
OPRM1, 81
OUD, *see* Opioid use disorder
Oxycodone, 57
OxyContin, 17, 53, 56, 57

P
Personality disorder, 38, 78
Peruvian Association of Therapeutic Communities (PTCA), 94
Pharmacotherapy, 10
Phenobarbital, 66
Phenytoin, 66
Phoenix House, 16
Pneumonia, 51
Post-traumatic stress disorder (PTSD), 27, 38
Prescription Behavior Surveillance System, 57
Prison TC, 117–119
cost-effectiveness, 123–124
vs. community TCs, 123
drug treatment programs, 120–121
efficacy, 119–123
Psychiatric comorbidity, 78
Psychotherapy, 40–41
PTSD, *see* Post-traumatic stress disorder

Q
QT interval prolongation, 67

R
Relapse prevention training, 10
Residential substance abuse treatment (RSAT), 117
Rifampicin, 66
R software, 143

S
San Patrignano (SanPa) therapy, 135–140
Seeking safety, 10
Self-detoxification methods, 64
Sertüner, F.W.A., 50
Services for addictions (SerD), 134
Service Standards for Therapeutic Communities, 35
Sexually transmitted diseases (STDs), 17
Short severity index, 142, 143
South American heroin, 27
SPSS software, 143
Staff burnout, 39
STDs, *see* Sexually transmitted diseases
Suboxone, 67
Substance-free lifestyle, 64
Substance use disorders (SUD), 26, 38
African Americans, 114
correctional setting, 114–115
DSM-IV criteria, 113

in prisons, 113
War on Drugs, 113
women, 38
Synanon, 24, 88
Synthetic opioids, 57

T

TCA, *see* Therapeutic Communities of America
Therapeutic communities (TC), 3, 75, 87
for addiction, 24–26
addiction workforce, 24–26
approach, 10–11
in Australasia, 93
Australasian Therapeutic Communities Association (ATCA), 93
characteristics of populations, 78–79
clinical supervision, 39
community based agencies, 10
components of, 32
correctional setting, 114–115
cost-effectiveness of, 123–124
drug treatment programs in prisons, 120–121
effectiveness of, 79
efficacy of prison, 119–123
European Federation of Therapeutic Communities (EFTC), 91
evidence-informed psychosocial treatment, 10
Federación Latinoamericana de Comunidades Terapéuticas (FLACT), 92–94
Federation of Therapeutic Communities in Asia (FTCA), 94–96
funding and planned duration of treatment, 13–14
hybridization of, 35–37
the international federations, 90
Italian model, 134–135
and the judicial system, 115–117
leadership in, 28
mechanism of efficacy, 80–81
movement, 89–90
opoid epidemic, 17–19
practice principles of, 33–35
in prison, 117–119
psychiatric conditions, 26–27
San Patrignano (SanPa), 135–138
structural components of, 32–35
Synanon, 88
theoretical framework, 12, 28–29
trauma-informed, 38–39
Treatment Communities of America (TCA), 90–91
treatment in correctional settings, 125–127
and the treatment gap, 81–82
Therapeutic Communities of America (TCA), 12
Therapeutic Community Essential Elements Scale Questionnaire (SEEQ), 35
Tobacco, 78
Tramadol, 69
Trans-theoretical model, 29
Treatment Communities of America (TCA), 90–91
Treatment resistant OUD, 76–78
community populations, 78–79
effectiveness of therapeutic communities, 79
therapeutic communities, 79
treatment gap, 81–82
Tuberculosis, 51
12-step groups, 10

U

Ultrarapid technique, 65
United Nations Office on Drugs and Crime (UNODC), 103

V
Vallmotorp, 89
Vincenzo Muccioli, 135, 136
Violent Crime Control and Law Enforcement Act, 1994, 117
Viral hepatitides, 2
Vivitrol, 69

W
War on Drugs, 113–114, 116
Winnicott's theory, 80
Wood, A., 50
World Federation of Therapeutic Communities (WFTC), 13, 92, 94–96

MIX
Papier aus verantwortungsvollen Quellen
Paper from responsible sources
FSC® C105338

If you have any concerns about our products,
you can contact us on
ProductSafety@springernature.com

In case Publisher is established outside the EU,
the EU authorized representative is:
Springer Nature Customer Service Center GmbH
Europaplatz 3, 69115 Heidelberg, Germany

Printed by Libri Plureos GmbH
in Hamburg, Germany